# Textbook on Clinical Research:
## A Guide for
## Aspiring Professionals and Professionals

### Second Edition

# Textbook on Clinical Research:
## A Guide for
## Aspiring Professionals and Professionals
## Second Edition

**Guru Prasad Mohanta**
**M. Pharm., Ph.D., FIC.**

Professor
Department of Pharmacy, Annamalai University,
Annamalai Nagar – 608 002, Tamilnadu.

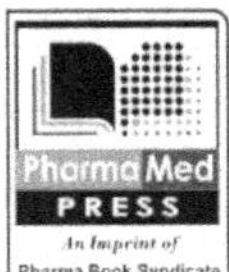

**PharmaMed Press**
*An imprint of Pharma Book Syndicate*
**A unit of BSP Books Pvt. Ltd.**
4-4-309/316, Giriraj Lane,
Sultan Bazar, Hyderabad - 500 095.

# *Dedicated to*

The Second Edition of this text is dedicated to the memory of my sister in law, Beena Mohanta, who left us early for heavenly abode. I must acknowledge her sincere goodwill and support which have been my strength for almost last three decades. She 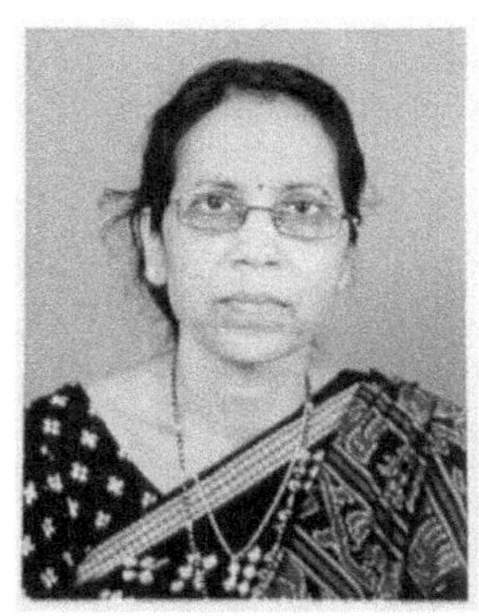 was a wonderful personality with all virtues and qualities one cannot forget. She was perhaps the most inspiring person for me and my family who used to feel happy even with our little success.

*-Author*

# Contents



**Chapter 1**

**Introduction**



**Chapter 2**

**Clinical Research in India**



**Chapter 3**

**Drug Development Process**

## Chapter 4

### Clinical Trials



## Chapter 5

### Ethical Issues in Clinical Research



## Chapter 6

### Good Clinical (Research) Practices (GCP) for Clinical Research in India

## Chapter 7

### Quality Assurance in Clinical Research



## Chapter 8

### Bioavailability and Bioequivalence Studies



## Chapter 9

### Data Management in Clinical Research ....................... 225



## APPENDICES



## Appendices of Schedule Y

Supplementary materials for this book will be available in
www.bspublications.net/9789352301669/

# Preface to Second Edition

"Either write something worth reading or do something worth writing".

- Benjamin Franklin

We have seen a remarkable changes in our view of how a clinical trial should be conducted atleast in India in the interest of preventing the exploitation of research participants and maintaining data integrity. This triggers the need of an updated text.

While the clinical research covers all types of investigation that address questions on the treatment, preparedness, diagnosis/ screening, or prognosis of disease or enhancement and maintenance of health; the clinical trials and bioequivalency testing are undoubtedly the most important ones. The clinical trials lead to discovery of new drug(s) or treatment. Inspite of tremendous growth in medical and pharmaceutical sciences, there have been huge gaps between the need and treatment options. It is necessary to promote such activities in the development of newer and safer interventional tools.

The clinical research in India has undergone  revolutionary changes in last couple of years.  There have been slow down of clinical research activities following Supreme Court's intervention. Following this, there are series of measures taken to streamline clinical trials and approval process in the larger interest of preventing patients' exploitation. However, a reversal trend has started in early 2016 with removal of restriction of number of trials per investigator, permitting trials in hospitals of less than 50 beds, and so on. These initiatives are viewed as to create conducive and appropriate environment for clinical trials in the country. 2017 is expected to see a comeback of clinical research activities.

The changes taken place after the publication of first edition necessitated the need of revising the text.  Hence, this updated second edition is brought. The edition has some new chapters too. Wish the new edition would continue to get the patronage from the readers.

I am grateful to my family: wife Reena, son Anupam and daughter Amrita for their encouragement and sparing me to completely revise the text. They have sacrificed family happy time for this work.  Mr. Anil Shah of PharmaMed Press requires special mention as without his personal interest it would have not been possible to have this revised text.

Last but not the least, I have taken all measures to make the upto date information available to the students, teachers and professionals. But if any lapse, it is my entire responsibility. Looking forward to receiving your feedback or suggestion for further refining the text.

**Guru Prasad Mohanta**

**E. mail: gpmohanta@hotmail.com**

# Preface to First Edition

"Arithmetic – is a bad master, but is a good servant. When this truth has been realized, the question of (the value of) medical records will appear in better perspective and the possibility of clinical research, not for the gifted few alone, but for all, will be admitted."

The Lancet

Clinical Research plays a major role in ensuring the availability of new drugs. The impact of globalization and rising cost of clinical research in developed countries has made all major pharmaceutical companies of the western world to look for off shoring the clinical research to other less developed countries including India. India becomes the favorite destination for clinical research due to basically cost competitiveness besides other advantages ranging from favorable regulatory aspects to easily available population to participate in the study.

The Indian clinical research industry has been growing fast and is estimated that its value would be around Rs. 8000 crore in 2010-2011 creating good employment opportunities for medical and pharmaceutical professionals. As the clinical research is a regulated area, specific norms – legal and ethical are stipulated in our statute. The people intending to be part of clinical research need to be qualified and well versed with the best practices in the industry. Adoption of Good Clinical Research Practice (GCP) ensures reliable evidence in establishing the safety and efficacy of medicines.

The present text attempts to provide the basics of clinical research relating to clinical trials, bioavailability and bioequivalence study. It covers the current scenario of clinical research industry, various aspects of clinical trials ranging from legal to ethical, bioequivalence study including GCP. In addition to these, the text gives the international requirements like ICH guidelines and USFDA regulations on clinical trials. The readers may find some aspects are repeated in different section or chapter, but are inevitable as they are essential part of that section or chapter. As the regulation and guidelines are dynamic in nature, the readers are encouraged to see the latest original regulation or guideline. Three important guidelines or regulations relating to clinical trials: ICH GCP, USFDA and EMEA can be downloaded from  www.bspublications.net/9789352301669

As the text is written in simple language, I believe the readers especially the student community will richly benefit. It has also attempted to cover the various aspects of the clinical research syllabus of Pharm. D. programme.

The preparation of the text would not have been easy without the support of my family: my wife Reena, son Anupam and daughter Amrita. I have no words to thank them. They are my support and strength. I express gratitude to two of my mentors:  Dr. R. Manavalan and Dr. P. K. Manna for their guidance and encouragement. The permission of Annamalai University Authority for writing the text is gratefully acknowledged. I do also express my sincere thanks to the World Health Organization for permitting me to use some of the materials from its publication.

Pharma Book Syndicate, Hyderabad, has done a good job of pursuing to write and publishing this book. Mr. Anil Shah of the publication deserves my appreciation and I thank him.

Though I have taken due care during the preparation of the text, there may be mistakes. I am entirely responsible for the same. However, I invite the readers' response and feed back for further improvement of the book. Their contribution will be gratefully acknowledged.

**Guru Prasad Mohanta**

**e-mail: gpmohanta@hotmail.com**

# Abbreviations

| | |
|---|---|
| ACET | Active Control Equivalence Trial |
| AD | Adverse Event |
| ALCOA | Attributable, Legible, Contemporaneous, Original and Accurate |
| ANOVA | Analysis of Variance |
| API | Active Pharmaceutical Ingredient |
| AUC | Area Under the Curve |
| BA | Bioavailability |
| BE | Bioequivalence |
| CA | Chromosomal Aberrations |
| CDSCO | Central Drug Standard Control Organization |
| CI | Confidence Interval |
| CIOMS | Council for International Organizations of Medical Sciences |
| COI | Conflict of Interest |
| CPU | Clinical Pharmacological Unit |
| CRA | Clinical Research Associate |
| CRO | Clinical Research Organization |
| CDMS | Clinical Data Management System |
| DMP | Data Management Plan |
| CRF | Case Report Form |
| CTRI | Clinical Trial Registry of India |
| DCGI | Drugs Controller General India |
| DGFT | Director General of Foreign Trade |
| DNA | Deoxyribonucleic Acid |
| DSMB | Drug Safety Monitoring Board |
| DTAB | Drugs Technical Advisory Board |
| ERB | Ethics Review Board |
| UNICEF | United Nations International Children Emergency Fund |
| UNAIDS | United Nations Programme on HIV/AIDS |
| $LD_{50}$ | Median Lethal Dose |
| EC | Ethics Committee |

| | |
|---|---|
| ECG | Electrocardiogram |
| EMA | European Medicines Agency |
| FDA | Food and Drugs Administration |
| FDC | Fixed Dose Combination |
| GCLP | Good Clinical Laboratory Practice |
| GCP | Good Clinical Practice |
| GLP | Good Laboratory Practice |
| GMP | Good Manufacturing Practices |
| GOI | Government of India |
| IC | Informed Consent |
| ICD | Informed Consent Document |
| ICF | Informed Consent Form |
| ICH | International Conference on Harmonization |
| ICMR | Indian Council for Medical Research |
| IDMA | Indian Drug Manufacturers Association |
| IDMC | Independent Data Monitoring Committee |
| IEC | Institutional Ethics Committee |
| IndEC | Independent Ethics Committee |
| IND | Investigational New Drug |
| INDA | Investigational New Drug Application |
| INN | International Nonproprietary Name |
| IP | Indian Pharmacopoeia |
| IPR | Intellectual Property Rights |
| IRB | Institutional Review Board |
| MCI | Medical Council of India |
| MLD | Minimum Lethal Dose |
| MNA | Micronucleus Assay |
| MTD | Maximum Tolerated Dose |
| MTP | Medical Termination of Pregnancy |
| NABH | National Board of Accreditation for Hospitals |
| NCE | New Chemical Entity |
| NIMS | National Institute of Medical Statistics |
| NOC | No Objection Certificate |
| OCR | Optical Character Recognition |

| | |
|---|---|
| OPPI | Organization of Pharmaceutical Producers of India |
| OTC | Over the Counter |
| OVI | Other Volatile Impurities |
| PI | Principal Investigator |
| PK | Pharmacokinetics |
| PSUR | Periodic Safety Update Report |
| QA | Quality Assurance |
| QC | Quality Control |
| RPM | Revolutions Per Minute |
| SAE | Serious Adverse Event |
| SD | Standard Deviation |
| SOP | Standard Operating Procedure |
| UTRN | Unique Trial Reference Number |
| WHO | World Health Organization |
| WMA | World Medical Association |

# CHAPTER 1

# Introduction

'I mean, shit, we learn by climbing over the bodies of humans.'
Murray Gardner, MD, University of California HIV Researcher

**After reading this chapter, you should be able to understand:**

- Clinical research – what and why? ;
- Different types of clinical research; and
- Prospects and Issues associated with clinical research.

Research is a quest for knowledge aimed at the discovery and interpretation of new knowledge.Clinical research, in simplest and broadest sense, is the research conducted on human beings leading to discovery of fact or information which increases the understanding of human health and disease. Clinical Research plays an important role in our efforts to maintain or promote health and combating diseases.

## What is Clinical Research?

Clinical research, a branch of health sciences, is defined as a well-planned, designed, executed, managed, and analysed study involving human beings (including materials of human origin such as tissues or behaviour) for testing the safety and efficacy of new drugs, devices or procedures in an attempt to use them for the benefit of mankind. It covers clinical trials, research in epidemiology, physiology, pathology, health education, outcomes and mental health. The ultimate objectives of the clinical research is to develop interventions to prevent, diagnose, treat illness and promote health.

People are often confused between the term 'clinical research' and 'medical care'. In medical care, the doctor develops a care plan for the patient (often in consultation with the patient) and the individual needs to follow. On the other hand, in clinical research, doctor and the individual need to follow a study protocol specifically designed for the purpose. It cannot be changed at doctor's or patient's wish.

Similarly, there are confusions between clinical research and clinical trials. Clinical trials are one type, perhaps most important type, of clinical research. Clinical research is a bigger domain and clinical trial is a subset of clinical research.

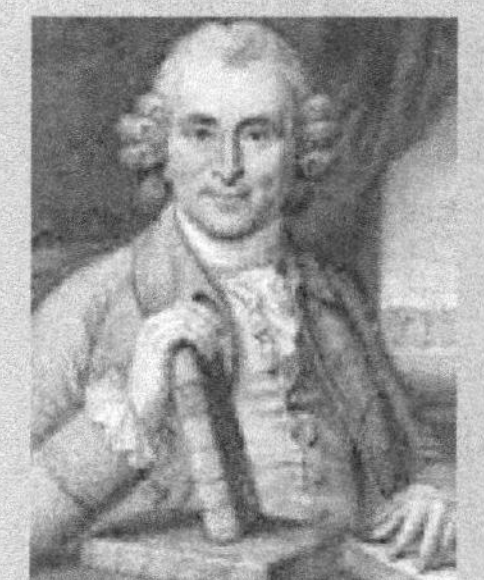

James Lind, Scottish doctor is credited to be the first scientist who performed clinical trial in 1747. Lind divided the 12 soldiers in the ship suffering from scurvy (symptoms are loose teeth, bleeding gums, and haemorrhage) into six pairs and gave different supplement to different group along with usual diet. Each pair's diet was supplemented by cider; sulphuric acid (elixir vitriol); vinegar; sea water; a mixture of nutmeg, garlic, mustard and tamarind in barley water; two oranges and one lemon daily. The pair receiving the oranges and lemon recovered within a week and back on duty. This led to the discovery of remedy of scurvy and Dr. Lind is recognized as father of clinical trial.

The clinical research has moved much beyond the general understanding of experiments or studies on living human beings. There are reports of experiments on 'living cadaver' or brain dead patients. The world's first clinical trial on the revival of brain dead patients in Uttarakhand town was reported recently.

## Why do we need Clinical Research?

Throughout the history of mankind, animal experimentations contributed immensely in our understanding of anatomy, physiology, pathology, microbiology, immunology, genetics etc. Scientists used animals in quest for knowledge. While animal experimentations are easy to perform, it is not possible to accurately predict or extrapolate the data from animals to humans. Besides, all human diseases cannot be reproduced in animals. World Health Organization's testing of typhoid vaccine in 1950s in Yugoslavia clearly demonstrates the difficulty of projection from animal experiment results to humans. Animal experiments showed that the alcohol killed and preserved vaccine was more effective than the heat killed phenol preserved vaccine. But the randomised controlled trials in humans showed the contrary results: Alcohol preserved vaccine effectiveness was found to be less than half of that of phenol preserved vaccine in preventing typhoid fever.

Hence, it is mandatory to do clinical research before a new drug or new treatment option is approved for mass use. Research in humans is our quest or aspiration to know and to advance our society. The purpose of clinical research is to find (list not exhaustive):

- New techniques for screening and diagnosing a disease;
- New drugs to introduce into market;
- New methods for surgery;
- New approach for therapy;
- New combinations of standard treatment;
- New techniques such as stem or gene therapy;
- Causes of illness.

## Types of Clinical Research

The common types of clinical research includes:

I.  Patient oriented research – Examples are: Mechanism(s) of human disease; Therapeutic intervention; Clinical trials; Development of new techniques.

II. Epidemiological and Behavioural research – Examples are: Distribution of diseases: Factors that affect health; How people make health related decision.

III. Outcome and Health Services research – Examples are: Identifying the most effective, and most efficient intervention, treatment and services.

The clinical research may be divided into two broad types: observational research and interventional research (or, experimental research). In observational research, researcher allows the nature to take its own course. The researcher just observes the natural course of events or outcomes and reports. On the other hand, in interventional or experimental research the researcher involves in active attempt to change a disease determinant or progress of the disease. The experiments are attempted to discover something unknown, or to test a hypothesis, or principle, but one cannot be sure of outcomes.

## Clinical Research Vs Clinical Trial

Clinical research is a research conducted with human subjects or materials of human origin. Clinical research is a broader term which includes both observational and experimental studies. But the clinical trials are one type of experimental clinical research. The clinical trial is a systematic study of pharmaceutical product or medical device in human subjects in order to assess their safety and / or efficacy. Clinical trials are done for various purposes and the most common types are (based on purpose):

(a) Prophylactic – Examples: testing of vaccines, contraceptives.

(b) Therapeutic – Examples: testing of new drugs, surgical techniques for efficacy.

(c) Safety trials – Examples: side effects of contraceptives.

(d) Risk factors trials – Examples: proving the aetiology of a disease by withdrawing the agent (smoking) through cessation.

The clinical trials are conducted under strict regulatory supervision.

## Scope of Clinical Research

As the clinical research including clinical trial aims to find out the suitability of a new drug, new drug product, or finding a new use of old drug, there would be continuing need of such research in the society. The pharmaceutical industries continue to invest on development of new drugs and so is the situation in medical device industries. New drugs are necessary not only for new diseases but also necessary for treatment of existing diseases like drug resistant tuberculosis. After laboratory investigation in experimental animals, it is necessary to conduct the safety and efficacy testing of a new treatment/drug through clinical trials before approval for mass use. Safety and efficacy are important criteria of any drug or drug products.

Persons qualified or trained in clinical research have good opportunities for employment in clinical trial industries or contract clinical research organizations as clinical research associates (CRAs) at different levels, clinical research monitor, clinical research manager, clinical research scientists, project manager, business development manager etc. As there are no fixed designations, the title of the posts may vary from industry to industry or from organization to organization. These clinical research professionals may be involved in all or some of these activities:

- Identifying and selecting investigator for the study;
- Coordinating with ethics committee for approval of the study;
- Coordinating with regulatory authority for seeking approval of the study;
- Visiting the investigation sites to assess their suitability to conduct the study;
- Organizing the investigators meeting and making presentations;
- Initiating, monitoring and closing of investigational sites;
- Training of site staff on Good Clinical Practice or other requirements of industry;

- Ensuring timely availability and distribution of investigational products;
- Developing protocol and case report forms;
- Preserving the study reports and all communications;
- Developing reports; and
- Preparing manuscript for publications.

## Issues in Clinical Research

The clinical research/clinical trial data are necessary for submission to regulatory authority seeking approval for marketing a new drug or drug product. Being human experiments, there is a necessity of preventing exploitation of research participants who may be healthy volunteers or patients. In order to protect the interest of research participants, there are strict rules and ethics guidelines which need to be adhered. The pharmaceutical industries often look at the poor countries for these studies. There are reports of violation of regulatory and ethical guidelines not only in poor countries but also in developed countries. More details of these guidelines and their violations are described in other chapters. There are issues even with quality of data generated during clinical research.

Many of drug research are either conducted or supported by pharmaceutical industries. Many of the clinical trials are reported to be with flawed design, flaw in data analysis, and misleading results. The results are cooked into conclusion as useful for boosting sales. The industries are often accused that they can make exploitation appear a noble purpose.

Irrespective of whether it is industry sponsored or non-industry based, the clinical research must follow the same standards. The research must be scientifically sound, follow basic ethical principles and ensures data of high quality.

In addition to misleading results, it is also alleged that many of the clinical research findings are not useful. The key features of useful research are outlined in the table:

| Feature | Questions to Ask |
| --- | --- |
| Problem base | Is there a health problem that is big/important enough to fix? |
| Context placement | Has prior evidence been systematically assessed to inform (the need for) new studies? |

*Table Contd....*

| Feature | Questions to Ask |
|---|---|
| Information gain | Is the proposed study large and long enough to be sufficiently informative? |
| Pragmatism | Does the research reflect real life? If it deviates, does this matter? |
| Patient centeredness | Does the research reflect top patient priorities? |
| Value for money | Is the research worth the money? |
| Feasibility | Can this research be done? |
| Transparency | Are methods, data, and analyses verifiable and unbiased? |
| Adopted from: IoannidisJPA(2016)WhyMostClinical ResearchIsNotUseful.PLoSMed13(6):e1002049. doi:10.1371/journal.pmed.1002049 ||

Though in broadest sense, the clinical research indicates that the research conducted on humans without involvement of any drug administration is also a type of clinical research (epidemiological research), the most important types of clinical research includes clinical trial and bioequivalence testing. The present text focusses on various aspects of clinical trial and bioequivalence.

## Key Points to Remember

- Clinical research is a well-planned, designed, executed, managed, and analysed study involving human beings (including materials of human origin such as tissues or behaviour) for testing the safety and efficacy of new drugs, devices or procedures in an attempt to use them for the benefit of mankind.
- Clinical trial is a type of clinical research aims to testing safety and efficacy of new drug/product/device.
- Clinical research needs to be conducted following regulatory and ethical standards to prevent exploitation of study participants and generate data of high quality.

James Lind was the scientist who had conducted the first clinical trial and is known as the father of clinical research.

# CHAPTER 2

# Clinical Research in India

"If clinical trials become a commercial venture in which self-interest overrules public interest and desire overrules science, then the social contract which allows research on human subjects in return for medical advances is broke".

Jonathan Quick, WHO, Director of Essential Drugs and Medicines Policy

**After reading this chapter, you should be able to:**

- Understand the scope of clinical research in India;
- Learn the recent changes in clinical research scenario like provision of compensation payment; and
- Perform a SWOT analysis on Prospects and Challenges of Clinical Trials in India.

The clinical trials and clinical research are often used interchangeably though they are different but overlapping. Clinical research is a broader term and clinical trial is just one type of clinical research. The present chapter focuses the two important aspects of clinical research: clinical trial and bioequivalence. Clinical trials are necessary to investigate the safety and efficacy of the promising drug or therapy and bioequivalence testing is to investigate the suitability of substitution among the various brands or between brand and innovator product. Bioequivalence ensures that the products are interchangeable.

The cost of drug development has steadily increased. The cost of developing a new drug was estimated to be US $ 2.6bn (2014) almost doubling the 2003 estimates of US $ 1.22bn. Clinical trial is one of the most important components in drug development process and costs around 70% of the total costs involved and requires about 7 years of research (out of 15 years time required for complete drug development process).

The increased focus on reducing the cost of drug development made the multinational pharmaceutical companies to look towards India and other economically weaker countries as a destination for clinical research. The multinationals spend around 40% of their R&D spending on clinical research. It is estimated that conducting clinical trial in India cost up to 60% less than in the US.

The 'Advantage India' (see the text box in the next page) outlines the reasons for shifting of focus for clinical trial from advanced countries to countries like India. The total number of clinical trials conducted in India was 221 in 2007 and increased to just over 700 trials in 2008 showing a growth of around 65%. There were reports of more than 100 companies conducting clinical trials in India. There were many foreign companies doing trial in India: Ranbaxy (now Sun), Astra Zeneca, Eli Lilly, GlaxoSmithKline, Pfizer, Johnson and Johnson, Novartis, Merck, Novo Nordisk etc. Even the Indian companies are not far behind the innovation initiatives. However, the initial growth of clinical trials in the country could not be sustained. The table below shows the declining trend of clinical trials:

| Year | Clinical Trials Approved |
|---|---|
| 2012 | 253 approved out of 480 applications |
| 2013 | 73 approved out of 207 applications |
| 2013 | 17 global clinical trials for conducting in India |
| 2014 | 87  global clinical trials for conducting in India |
| 2015 August | 43 global clinical trials for conducting in India |

Some estimate shows that about 1.4% of clinical trials conducted globally are being done in India. In spite of being the home of one-sixth of the world population and with one – fifth of the global disease burden, the clinical research opportunities have slowed down. India is lagging behind the countries like Korea, Taiwan, and Japan.

## Clinical Trials

**Advantage India:**

1. **Very large population with diverse ethnic group** – Many are not previously exposed to similar medicines. This makes the results more reliable.

2. *Physical infrastructure:* Large number of hospitals and laboratories available. The hospitals and laboratories are in the process of getting accreditation for getting global acceptance. In the country there are more than 700,000 speciality hospital beds.

3. *Trained manpower:* Large number of medically qualified persons (more than 200 medical colleges), pharmacy qualified persons, nurses and others. Little training would make them familiar with legal and ethical issues.

4. *Favourable regulation:* Drugs and Cosmetics Act and the Rules amended to allow simultaneously clinical trial as done in other countries. Exemption of provision of registration for import of materials for clinical trial, no import duty on clinical trial supplies, GCP and ethical guidelines in place are on par with International guidelines and favourable patent law.

5. *Government support:* Tax concession for R&D activities, exemption of service tax.

6. *Recruiting patients easier:* Recruiting 200 patients in US for one year study requires approximately 30 months while this can be done in less than half of the time. In India patients are ignorant of their rights, patients completely rely on doctors, monitoring mechanism is lax are added advantages.

7. *Lower cost:* Lower wages to key personnel involved in clinical trial and data monitoring, clinical research assistants, project management, clinical data management and biostatisticians.

8. *Data Management skill:* Good IT helps in managing large pool of data generated during clinical trials.

9. *Use of English:* As the medium of instruction in professional programme is English, all the professionals for clinical research would have good English language skills. It not only helps with communication but also in data management.

10. *Few drop outs:* In the eagerness to get good quality of medical care, the subjects are less likely to leave study. Thus there are less drop outs.

11. *Patent regime* is in compliance with International requirements.

**Concerns:**

1. Data Integrity becomes a big issue.

2. Lack of trained manpower especially doctors with GCP experience. There is need of trained nurses, biostatisticians, monitors, auditors, bio-analytical scientists, pharmacokinetic experts etc.

3. Lack of sufficient number of accredited laboratories for analysis of samples.

4. Exploitation of patients: The patients are unaware of their rights. Many are illiterate. Lack of compensatory measures. No guarantee of post trial access to medicines.

5. Poor implementation of regulation: Lack of staff in drugs control department, often they are not trained to monitor the trial. Of late some initiatives are made to recruit more staff and train them with GCP guidelines for inspecting clinical trial sites.

6. Ethics committees are often not constituted properly nor do they function independently and in transparent way. Ethics committee members are not even aware of the need of compensation to participants if they suffer an injury because of trial.

7. Permission to conduct clinical trial takes longer time: Approval for conducting clinical trial takes a minimum of eight months where as in countries like Canada, USA, the Netherlands, UK etc. it takes just one month.

The liberalised clinical trial guidelines of 2005 led to the growth of clinical trials and at the same time the participating volunteers or patients were reported to have been exploited. The investigators were found to have violated the ethical standards in not obtaining patients' consent and not compensating to those who suffered adverse side effects. The clinical trials were conducted on vulnerable groups like children and patients with learning disability. The Indian legislation, Drugs and Cosmetics Act and the Rules, requires that DCGI permission is required for conducting clinical trials but there is no provision for punishment of any kind for violating guidelines. The law just empowers the DCGI to suspend or stop the trial midway and order an enquiry. The Parliamentary Standing Committee of Health and Family Welfare Ministry came down heavily on the functioning of CDSCO with respect to irregularity in clinical trial approval and conductance (August 2013). Following the receipt of several complaints and public interest litigation, the Supreme Court stepped in 2013 ordering to stop all clinical trials until a mechanism is in place to monitor them. Following the Supreme Court's ruling, 162 trials approved by the DCGI have been put on hold. This led the Government to take a series of measures to strengthen the regulatory measures in public interest. These are:

- Constitution of expert committee for examining the trial proposal: a three tier system is made in place;
- Mandatory audio-visual recording of the process of obtaining written informed consent for each trial subject;
- Stringent compensation guidelines for payment to clinical trial participants who suffer from injury;
- Need of disclosure of contract between the sponsor and investigator with regard to financial support, fees, honorarium and payments in kind to be paid to the investigator;
- Provision of regulatory inspection of clinical trial sites;
- Introducing Drugs and Cosmetics (Amendment) Bill 2013 in Parliament containing penal provision for violation of clinical trial procedures and provision for payment of compensation and ethics committee;
- Restricting the number of clinical trials to the investigator to just three; and
- Mandatory registration of ethics committees and their accreditation.

In addition, the Government of India established an expert committee, Ranjit Roy Chaudhury panel, to advice on policy guidelines for approval of new drugs, clinical trials and banning of drugs. You may refer the box given in next pages to know the salient features of the report.

A SWOT analysis of current clinical trial scenario is given in the tabular column.

| Strength | Weakness | Opportunities | Threats |
| --- | --- | --- | --- |
| • Large population with diverse ethnic group and disease burden. | • No regulatory provision to punish violating organizations. | • Steps to carry easy business in India (trial norms are liberalised – removing restriction on the number of trial per investigator, empowering ethics committees on site selection etc.) | • Regulatory Challenges – Uncertainty due to several temporary measures taken. The Rules are yet to be amended. |

**Table *Contd...***

| Strength | Weakness | Opportunities | Threats |
|---|---|---|---|
| • Large number of hospitals and laboratories with excellent infrastructure. | • No adequate mechanism to monitor clinical trials and to safeguard the participating volunteers or patients from exploitation. | • Removal of phase lag and permission to conduct simultaneously phase - 1 trials with rest of the world. | • Misconception about human studies. |
| • Huge pool of qualified and trained human resources. | | • Mandatory Registration and Accreditation of Ethics Committees redress the usual quality issues in clinical trials. | • Lack of awareness about the benefit of participating in clinical trials. |
| • Lower cost of a trial. | | • Adequate compensatory provision may encourage people to participate in the trials. | • Data integrity is an issue – there are reports of falsification and manipulation of data by the clinical research organizations |

**Salient Points of Professor Ranjit Roy Chaudhury Expert Committee Report [relating to clinical trials], July 2013:**

1. Clinical trials are to be conducted only at accredited sites by an accredited investigator and the study should be approved by an accredited ethics committee. The trials which satisfy these requirements will only be acceptable by DCGI.

2. A Central Accreditation Council should be set up to oversee the accreditation of institutes, clinical investigators and institute ethics committees. Selection of assessors for accreditation and of experts to review new drug applications and other purposes will be made by a blind randomized procedure from a Roster of Experts. This Roster will be prepared after a nationwide search of appropriate experts and approval by the Technical Review Committee. The selection will have built-in safeguards for gender sensitivity and geographical representation.

3. The pharmaceutical houses are required to identify the centres out of the rosters established for conducting the clinical treals.

4. It is necessary to establish expertise-based Technical Review Committee to ensure speedy clearance of applications without compromising on quality of data and rules and regulations. The Committee would be assisted as required by appropriate subject experts selected from the Roster of Experts.

5. An informed consent from each participant is a mandatory prerequisite for a clinical trial. Where consent is received from guardian for persons with diminished capacity, the consent given should be witnessed by an independent person who also has to sign the informed consent document. Audio-visual recording of consent process should be undertaken and the documents are to be preserved adhering to the principle of confidentiality.

6. In the event of any adverse effect (AE) or serious adverse effect (SAE), the sponsor/investigator will be responsible for providing medical treatment and care to the patient at his/their cost till the resolution of the *AE/SAE*. This is to be given irrespective of whether the patient is in the control group, placebo group, standard drug treatment group or the test drug administered group.

7. a. Compensation related to injury or death due to unrelated causes: No compensation is required to be paid. In all other cases of injury, death / disability, compensation is to be paid to the participant or legal heir.

   b. Compensation needs to be paid to the trial participant even if an anomaly related to drug is discerned at a later stage in India or abroad.

   c. Trial in terminally ill patients: Compensation needs to be paid if the IEC is of the opinion that there is an increase in SAEs or life expectancy is severely curtailed. However, compensation may not be given if the primary end-point is death as per the clinical trial protocol.

8. Compensation needs to be paid to the placebo group too if they suffer from SAE.

9. No compensation is needed in case of therapeutic inefficiency.

10. IEC should be empowered to decide the cause of injury or death.

11. There must be strong provision for ancillary care to cater for patients suffering from any other Illness during the trial.

12. Academic research may be approved by Institute Ethics Committee. No need of DCGI Approval.  However, if trial is for

new drug or new use of an existing drug, DCGI approval is necessary.

13. The Central Government, State Governments and academic institutions should create fund to encourage academic research (non-pharmaceutical company sponsored research). The fund may be used for paying compensation.

14. Phases I to IV clinical trials is a must for all new entities developed in India to be marketed in India.

15. All NCEs/NMEs undergoing clinical trials anywhere can also undergo parallel Phase II and Phase III trials in India after carrying out a safety assessment through Phase I trials.

16.

    (a) Drugs already in the market in well-regulated countries with good post-marketing surveillance (PMS) for more than four years and which have a satisfactory report may be granted marketing licence, subject to strict PMS for four to six years. The period of four years may be reduced or waived off in cases where no therapy or only palliative therapy is available, or in national healthcare emergencies.

    (b) First-time generics manufactured in India will undergo bridging Phase III trials and bioequivalence (BE) studies in humans.

    (c) BE studies in humans should be undertaken in subsequent generics along with strict PMS.

    (d) Similar biologics (biosimilars) need to undergo both pre-clinical development and bridging Phase III clinical trials as per Department of Biotechnology (DBT)- Central Drugs Standard Control Organization (CDSCO) guidelines.

17.

    (a) Where new chemical entities (NCEs)/ new biological entities (NBEs) or new drug substances or their generic drugs or similar biologics are to be introduced in India, bioavailability (BA)/BE studies in patients should be done preferably as a part of the clinical trial.

    (b) BA and BE studies of new drug substances discovered abroad and not marketed in India should be conducted in India.

    (c) BA and BE studies once conducted with a generic should not be repeated for just export purposes.

18. Approval of clinical trials should be given within three months of proper documentation required for review.

19. At any point of time, the representative of the pharmaceutical house or investigator shall have the right of dialogue with an officer of the CDSCO regarding the application on payment of a fee for such consideration.

20. Information technology is to be explored at all steps of a clinical trial to ensure total transparency in the system. From the first step when the application is placed at the single window, till the final approval is received, every step will be recorded and made available in the public domain.

21. For State level Monitoring these activities are suggested: Joint monitoring with CDSCO staff, coordination and information sharing, and training of state regulatory staff.

The pragmatic shift has raised the international concern and the regulatory changes have forced many multinational companies to withdraw their clinical trials causing the declining trend. The US National Institute of Health (NIH) announced suspension of its 40 clinical trials because of new requirements.

Realising the need of efforts to promote clinical trials as a part of easy doing business in India and as well the need of new drug discovery to meet the unmet treatment need, the Government of India has initiated several steps. They are meant to strengthening regulatory scenario to protect the interest of the clinical trial participants while easing the provision for doing business. Some of these are:

- Provision of online submission of clinical trial applications;

- Provision of pre-submission meeting between stake holders and drug regulators in a bid to enable technical deliberations before submitting the final application seeking clinical trial approval;

- Reviewing and approval timeline for all types approval is limited to six months;

- Pre-clinical testing waiver if the new molecule is already approved outside India (no need of animal testing);

- Not limiting the number of trials per investigator (limit of restricting three trials per investigator is removed). Ethics Committee is empowered to decide how many trials an investigator can take at a time based on the risks and complexity of the trial;

- Planning to revise the requirement that the trial must be conducted at site with more than 50 hospital beds;

- Empowering Ethics Committees to add trial sites and investigators without the need of obtaining no objection certificate from DCGI. The company needs to inform the changes to DCGI;

- Liberalising academic clinical research – there is no need of DCGI approval for conducting academic clinical research in respect of approved drug or product if (i) the trial is approved by RC and (ii) data generated is not intended for submission to regulatory authority;

- Balanced compensation guidelines: In case of injury occurring to the subject during the clinical trial, free medical management shall be given as long as required or until such time it is established that the injury is not related to the clinical trial, whichever is earlier [the previous guideline provided free medical treatment to these patients by sponsors irrespective of whether the impairment was related or not related to a clinical trial]. In case, there is no permanent injury, the quantum of compensation shall be commensurate with the nature of the injury and loss of wages of the subjects.

- Provision of parallel application to the review committee on Genetic Manipulation and DCGI for seeking approval of trial for r-DNA derived drugs like insulin, monoclonal antibodies etc.

- Extending the validity of Bioavailability / Bioequivalence Study centres, and bio-analytical laboratories from one year to three years.

All these initiatives are likely to help regaining of 'Advantage India' position for clinical research.

## Key Points to Remember

- Clinical trials in India has undergone a revolutionary changes in last couple of years.

- Following the amendment of schedule Y in 2005 and other favorable conditions such as acceptance of product patent, duty free import of clinical trial materials boosted the clinical research in India. The total number of clinical trials conducted in India was 221 in 2007 and increased to just over 700 trials in 2008 showing a growth of around 65%. There were reports of unethical practices and exploitation of patients.

- There were several measures taken by the Government after the Supreme Court's direction to stop the clinical trials until a suitable mechanism to monitor is in place. These measures are to bring more transparency and accountability. Ranjit Roy Chaudhury Panel's report is the guiding force.

- Some of the measures taken by the Government are: Restricting the number of clinical trials to an investigator is three, mandatory registration of ethics committee, formula for deciding the compensation payment to research participants in case of trial related injury etc.

- The above strict measures have caused shifting of clinical trial business from India to other countries.

- In order to ease clinical research as a part of promoting environment for easy doing business, several measures are initiated including removing the restriction of number of trials to an individual investigator, empowering the ethics committee to take decision of the site and investigator, time bound disposal of trail applications, extending the validity period of approval of BA/BE centres and bio-analytical centres from one year to three years, etc.

- Academic research with approved drug are exempted from taking DCGI approval provided the research is approved by Ethics Committee and the data generated are not for seeking regulatory approval.

- While 'Advantage India' factors like Large population with diverse ethnic group and disease burden, large number of hospitals and laboratories with excellent infrastructure, huge pool of qualified and trained human resource, and lower cost of a trial make the India a favourable destination for clinical research, there are many concerns too including the quality of data. Many companies are under regulatory scanner.

- The Government's policy to promote clinical research in the country while taking adequate measures to protect the interest of research or study participants and ensuring quality data perhaps will revive the clinical research business.

# CHAPTER 3

# Drug Development Process

"If we take care in the beginning, the end will take care of itself"

**After reading this chapter, you should be able to understand or know:**

- Need and Methods used in drug discovery;
- Various phases of drug discovery: journey from new drug molecule to new drug application; and
- Concept of testing the drug in human subjects

Drugs are perhaps the most important therapeutic interventions in modern health care. Development of new drugs is always a prime concern for research based pharmaceutical industries. Though the plant materials have been used as reservoir of potential drugs through the history, the new drugs may be discovered from a variety of natural sources or synthesized in the laboratory. They may be discovered by accident. But at present the drugs development requires many years of tireless pursuit. Genetic engineering and biotechnological advancement provides new platform for drug development process. Molecular level understanding of the disease process further streamlines the process of drug discovery in identifying the target. As a whole, the process and time course from drug discovery to marketing is a lengthy and tedious process. It takes about 10-15 years to develop one new medicine from the time it is discovered to when it is available for treating patients. The average cost is estimated to be USD 2.6 billion (2014).

## Approaches to Drug Discovery

There is always a need for developing new drugs. Old drugs become ineffective especially with development of microbial resistance. Because of non-availability of new antibiotics, treatment of resistant tuberculosis becomes extremely difficult. Peoples' longevity has increased and there is need of treatment of age related illnesses. Even the new diseases are emerging for which no treatment available. Remedy of Zika virus infection is a distanced dream. Chikungunya and Dengue are reported to have taken several lives in India just because there is no effective treatment. The treatment available for Hepatitis C becomes extremely unaffordable. Alternative affordable treatment must be made available in the interest of public health.

Previously the drugs were discovered through identifying the active principles from traditional remedies (Artemisinin for malaria) or serendipity (Penicillin first antibiotic which revolutionised the treatment of infections). The process of drug discovery over the years has undergone a paradigm shift from serendipity to a more rational way of process. Rational approach involves the design of a compound of a particular activity. Irrespective of drug discovery method, the drug discovery in general begins with identifying a promising molecule (a lead compound) that could become a drug. The lead compound is a prototype chemical compound that has a fundamental desired biologic or pharmacologic activity. There are several ways to find a lead compound: Nature, *De novo,* High – throughput screening, Biotechnology. High throughput screening is a robotic process used to identify the 'hit compounds' which are further investigated to know their physical, chemical or biological properties. Hit compounds with suitable physicochemical and biological properties are lead compounds. The lead compound may not possess all desired features of a successful drug. Thus they are modified to produce analogues with additional or different functional chemical groups, altered ring structure, or different chemical configurations. The lead compounds go through a series of tests to provide an early assessment of the safety of lead compounds. The pharmacokinetics and toxicity study of each lead compound are performed in living cells, in animals or via computational models. Currently much emphasis is on identifying the cause and process of a disease and then designing molecules capable of interfering with that process. Most diseases arise from a biochemical imbalance, an abnormal proliferation cells, an endogenous deficiency, an exogenous chemical toxin or an invasive pathogen.

Modern methods of drug discovery uses the softwares obtained from Accelerys, FlexX, and Schrodinger etc. They are called Computer Aided Drug Design. More details are beyond the scope of this text.

## Six Basic Approaches to Drug Discovery

1. Identification of new drug target: A target is usually a single gene, a gene product or a molecular mechanism that has been identified on the basis of genetic analysis or biological observations. The completion of human genome project has resulted in identifying as many as 7000 targets.
2. Drug design based on biological mechanisms, drug receptor structure, and drug structure. This includes CADD.
3. Chemical modification of known drug.
4. Screening of known products: Natural products, peptides, nucleic acids are exploited.
5. Biotechnology and Cloning.
6. Combination of known drugs (Fixed Dose Combinations) either to improve therapeutic efficacy or reduce toxicity or reduce the incidence of resistance or repositioning a known drug for new indication.

The lead compounds that survive the initial safety testing are then optimized or altered in an attempt to make them more effective and safer.

With one or more optimized compounds in hand, it is necessary now to test them extensively for safety and efficacy both in living cell cultures and animal model. This phase of evaluation is pre-clinical testing. The pre-clinical testing results are the foundation for clinical testing on human beings. The clinical testing requires the regulatory approval.

## Preclinical Testing

The primary aim of pre-clinical (animal) testing is to obtain basic information on the drug's effects that may be used to predict safe and effective use in humans. Unfortunately, useful animal models are not available for every human disease. There are species difference between animals and humans too. Hence, it is essential that the drug needs testing in human beings too before being approved for marketing (general use). Accordingly, the objective of animal testing is to generate all data that satisfy all requirements before a new compound is deemed fit to be tested for the first time in humans.

This pre-clinical testing can be divided into two broad categories: pharmacological testing including pharmacokinetic testing and toxicological testing.

### (a) Pharmacological Screening

The prospective drug substances are tested for biological activity to assess their potential for developing as drugs. The work basically involves pharmacological and toxicological screening of the substance to determine whether the substance has effectiveness and a reasonable safety profile. A stepwise progress through increasingly sophisticated evaluation based on test compound's success in prior studies is followed:

- *Molecular Level Study:* The prospective substance is studied for its selectivity (affinity) for various receptors and its activity against selective enzyme systems. Cell membrane fractions from organs or cultured cells, cloned receptors, sympathetic nerves, adrenal glands, purified enzymes, liver etc. are used. Example: Receptor binding study can be performed in cell membrane fractions from organs or cultured cells.

- *Cellular Level Study:* The use of cell and tissue culture and computer programmes that simulate human and animal system are increasingly used to assess the pharmacological action (toxicity as well). Testing through these systems have reduced the dependence on the use of animals. Isolated tissues are also equally helpful in identifying the substance's activity and selectivity. Isolated tissues like blood vessels, heart, lung, ileum of rat or guinea pig are used. The study of antibacterial agent in bacterial culture, effect on vascular contraction and relaxation in isolated tissues and effect on other smooth muscles in isolated tissues are few examples.

- *Whole Animal Study:* Whole animal studies are generally necessary to determine the effect of prospective substance on organ systems and disease models. These studies are generally reserved for testing substances that have demonstrated reasonable potential in *in vitro* testing. Where possible, studies on disease models are to be performed. A number of animal models are available to mimic certain human diseases and are effectively used in screening. The examples in this category include: study of antihypertensive effects in hypertensive rats, central nervous system effects like degree of sedation, muscle relaxation in mouse or rat.

The pharmacological testing also ensures that the drug does not produce any potential hazardous or serious unwanted effects like bronchoconstriction, changes in blood pressure etc.

The pharmacokinetic testing is done to determine: the extent and rate of absorption from various routes of administration, including the one intended for human use; the rate of distribution of the drug though the body and the site(s) and duration of drug's residence; the primary and secondary rate, site and mechanism of drug metabolism in the body, chemistry and pharmacology of any metabolites; and the proportion of administered dose eliminated from the body and its rate and route of elimination. In these studies, a minimum of two animal species are employed (rodent and dog).

### (b) Toxicological Evaluation

No drug is safe, at all doses. All drugs are toxic at some dose. Toxicity is the most difficult drug property to adequately evaluate, because it could be species specific, organ specific, and could involve multiple host factors and chronic dosing regimens and all of which cannot be adequately modelled experimentally. Though toxicity data on animals can not be completely extrapolated to humans because of reasons like species variation, different dose-response relationship, immunological differences etc., it is necessary to test the test drug first in several species of animals. The greater the number of animal species tested that demonstrate a toxic effect, the greater the chance the effect will be seen in humans.

The toxicity studies are under taken to determine the test drug's: potential for toxicity with short term (acute toxicity) and long term use (long term toxicity); potential for specific organ toxicity; mode, site and degree of toxicity; dose – response relationship for low, high and intermediate doses over a specified time; gender, reproductive or teratogenic toxicities; and potential for carcinogenic and genotoxicity.

Most animal testing is done on small animals, usually rodents (mouse, rat) for reasons of cost, availability, requirement of less quantity drug, ease of administration and experience with drug testing in these species. However, in final studies, two or more animal species are used. The test drugs are studied at various dose levels to determine effects, potency and toxicity. The following toxicity studies are recommended by regulatory authorities:

(a) *Acute (Short – Term) Toxicity Studies*: The prospective drugs substance is administered at various dose levels to find the largest single dose that will not produce a toxic effect; the dose level at which severe toxicity occurs; and intermediate toxicity levels. During this short term study the animals are observed and compared with controls for eating and drinking habits, weight change, toxic effects, psychomotor changes, and any other signs of untoward effects, usually over a 30 days post dosing period. The biological samples are tested to detect changes in clinical chemistry and other changes that could indicate toxicity. In the event of death, histological and pathological data should be evaluated on the basis of dose – response, gender, age, intraspecies and interspecies findings against control.

(b) *Sub-acute (Sub-chronic) Toxicity Studies*: This involves giving the prospective drug substance daily for a minimum period of two weeks at three or more dosage levels to two animal species. This study is useful generating evidence to support the initial administration of a single dose in human clinical testing. Generally one tenth of the highest non toxic dose in mg per kg body weight is the initial dose in human.

(c) *Chronic Toxicity Studies:* The animal studies of three to six months is required if the tested drug is intended to be given for one week or more in humans. For drugs intended to be given for chronic illness, animal studies for one year or longer is required.

The comparative data of test and control during sub-chronic and chronic studies: duration of treatment, observed effects, mortality, body weight changes, food and water consumption, physical examination, haematology, clinical chemistry, organ weights, gross pathology, histopathology, urine analysis etc. are to be generated.

**(d)** *Reproduction Studies:* The effects of the prospective drug substance in reproductive performance are studied in mammalian species to assess fertility and mating behaviour; early embryonic, prenatal, and post natal development; multigenerational effects; and teratology.

The maternal parents, foetus, neonates, and weaning offspring are evaluated for anatomic abnormalities, growth, and development. Though the same species used in other toxicity studies are used here, but a second mammalian species is necessary for embryo toxicity. In the study, high dose is selected based on previous study with lower dosage in descending sequence.

**(e)** *Carcinogenicity Studies:* These studies are usually carried out in a limited number of rat and mouse strains for which there is reasonable information on spontaneous tumour incidence. The high dose to be used for the study should be maximum tolerated dose to elicit signs of minimal toxicity without significantly altering the animal's normal life span by effects other than carcinogenicity.

In a long term study, the survived animals are killed and studied at defined time and data on causes of death (other than killing), tumour incidence, type and site, and findings of necropsy.

**(f)** *Genotoxicity (Mutagenicity) Studies:* These studies are performed to determine the effects of the prospective drug substance on genetic stability and mutations in bacteria (Ames Test) or mammalian cells in culture, dominant lethal test and clastogenicity in mice.

In addition to the above studies some quantitative estimates are desirable: the maximum dose at which a specified toxic effect is not seen (no effect dose) and the smallest dose that is observed to kill any experimental animal (minimum lethal dose). Because of increased concern on use of animals for generating valid pre-clinical data, cell and tissue culture *in vitro* methods are increasingly used, but their predictive value is limited.

The requirements for detail data on animal testing are given in Appendix III and Appendix IV of schedule Y of Drugs and Cosmetics Rules. The readers can refer the same in Appendix to Schedule Y.

## Development of Chemical and Pharmaceutical Information

The appendix 1 of Drugs and Cosmetics Rules Y specifies the data under Chemical and Pharmaceutical Information subheading required to be submitted with the application to conduct clinical trials. The importance of each component is narrated briefly. However, to know more how the parameter is to be determined, the readers are encouraged to see other texts.

Once the prospective drug substance crossed the pharmacologic and toxicology evaluation in animals, it becomes necessary to generate data on chemical and physical properties that are useful for developing stable and effective pharmaceutical formulation (product). This part of the study is intended generating information relating to composition, manufacture, stability and controls used for manufacturing the drug substance and the product.

This information is assessed to ensure that the sponsor or the company has the ability to produce and supply consistence batches of the drug substance. The data are reviewed to evaluate the manufacturing and processing procedures for a drug to ensure that the drug substance is adequately reproducible and stable. If the drug is either unstable or not reproducible, then validity of any clinical testing would be undermined because one would not know what was really being used in the patients and the studies may pose significant risks to patients.

1. **Information on Active Ingredients:** The drug substance is basically a chemical and is identified by several names. The following names are the most important: Chemical Name and Generic Name (or INN). The chemical name describes every part of the drug substance's molecular structure, so that it describes only that substance (compound) and no other. The Generic Name is the shortened name of the chemical, also known as non-proprietary name. International Non-Proprietary Name (INN) is internationally recognized shortened name of

pharmaceuticals and also called generic name. World Health Organization has designed the procedure for coining INN.

2. **Physicochemical Data:**

   ***Chemical Name and Structure:*** Empirical Formula and Molecular Weight. The empirical formula indicates the number and relationship of the atoms in the molecule. Molecular weight is the characteristic of the compound and even validates the empirical formula.

   ***Physical Properties:*** Description, Solubility, Rotation, Partition Coefficient, Dissociation Constant.

   Though most of the drug substances are solid in nature, the use of liquids and gases as drugs are not uncommon. The purity of a chemical substance is essential for its identification. The physical description includes physical form, whether crystalline or amorphous, properties observed under microscopic examination such as particle size, shape etc.

   Solubility especially aqueous solubility is important for therapeutic activity. A drug must first be in solution before being absorbed into the system. Relatively insoluble compounds often exhibit incomplete or erratic absorption. Data on solubility helps formulation too.

   Specific rotation is a characteristic of the compound. Even the pharmacologic activity depends on whether the optically active compound is dextro or laevo rotatory form or a racemic mixture.

   The partition coefficient of the compound in a solvent system is again a characteristic property. The partition coefficient of substance between octanol – water system is a good indicator of drug absorption *in vivo*.

   Dissociation Constant is an indication of extent of dissociation or ionization which is highly dependent on pH of the medium containing the drug. It has good influence in formulation and pharmacokinetic parameter of the drug. Often the pH of the vehicle is adjusted to ensure certain level of ionization for solubility and stability. The extent of ionization of a drug has strong effect on its extent of absorption, distribution and elimination.

3. **Analytical Data:** Elemental Analysis, Mass Spectrum, NMR Spectra, IR Spectra, UV Spectra, Polymorphic Identification:

The elemental analysis confirms the molecular formula of the drug substance. The mass spectroscopy, NMR spectroscopy, IR spectroscopy, and UV spectroscopy are used to establish the identity of the compound. The acidic or basic nature of the compound can be predicted from functional groups. The data may also be useful in developing an analytical method.

The polymorphic form, whether crystalline or amorphous, of a drug substance is an important consideration on formulation. The different polymorphic forms exhibit different physicochemical properties, stability and bioavailability.

4. **Complete Monograph Specification including Identification, Identity/ Quantification of impurities, Enatiomeric purity, Assay**:

The identification test for the compound is essential to ensure authenticity when new batch of substance is manufactured or obtained from other source. The identification tests include chemical tests, melting point etc.

Impurities that may arise in the synthetic process used to manufacture drug substance may get access to the final product. They may be toxic. Hence it is essential to identify and quantify the impurities present in drug substance.

Enatiomeric purity refers to the presence of extent of active isomer. Active isomer may get converted to the inactive form with time. Thus the proportion of active isomer in drug substance sample is important.

Assay value of the drug substance signifies the purity of the drug substance.

5. **Validations:** Assay method, Impurity estimation method, and Residual solvent /other volatile impurities estimation method.

The validated analytical methods are required to be established and they should be used for assay, estimation of impurities and residual solvent or impurities in drug substance. The validated analytical method ensures that the procedure will give reproducible and reliable results. The validated analytical method helps establishing the specifications for quality of drug substance.

6. **Stability Studies:** Final release specification, Reference standard characterization, Material safety data sheet.

The physico-chemical stability of drug substance is critical to formulating a successful final product. The stability data is essential for formulation, designing the processing condition, and storage condition to be employed.

The reference standard refers to an authenticated uniform material with adequate purity that is intended for use in specified chemical and physical tests, in which its properties are compared with the properties of the sample in consideration. It is necessary to generate adequate data on reference substance to characterise it so that it can be used as reference for identification or determining purity of the drug substance in consideration.

7. **Data on Formulation:** Dosage form, Composition, Master manufacturing formula, Details of the formulation (including inactive ingredients), In process quality control check, Finished product specifications, Excipient compatibility study, Validation of the method, Comparative evaluation with International Brands(s) or approved Indian Brand(s) (if applicable), Stability evaluation in market intended pack at proposed storage conditions, Packing specifications, and Process validation

The product intended for clinical trial must be manufactured complying with Good Manufacturing Practice requirements. The data described above helps the regulatory authority to assess and ensure that:

- There would be consistency between and within the batches of investigational product.
- There would be consistency between investigational product and future commercial product.
- The subjects would not be exposed to poor quality product.

Selection of appropriate dosage form for clinical trial is important. It may be possible that dosage form employed in early clinical trial is different from the anticipated final formulation. However, the product intended for use in phase – III trial should be similar to the final product.

If there are significant differences between the product used in clinical trial and the final product intended for marketing, adequate data must be generated to demonstrate that the final product is equivalent to the product used in clinical trial in terms of bioavailability and stability.

## Investigational New Drug Application (INDA)

The INDA is required to be submitted to Drug Regulatory Authority before initiation of Clinical Trial. The INDA can be submitted by the sponsor but may employ CRO to conduct the actual studies. The Appendix 1 of Schedule Y of Drugs and Cosmetics Rules specifies the data required to be submitted along with the application to conduct clinical trial.

The INDA can be submitted for one or more phases of clinical investigation (described later in the chapter). The INDA is reviewed to ensure the protection of rights and safety of the human subjects and that the investigational plan is sound and allows evaluation of safety and effectiveness on approval.

### US FDA Requirement (Contents INDA)

- Name, address, and telephone number of the sponsor of the drug.
- Name and title of the person responsible for monitoring the conduct and progress of the investigation.
- Names and titles of the persons responsible for the review and evaluation of information relevant to safety of the drug.
- Name and address of any CRO involved in the study.
- Identification of the phase or phases of clinical investigation to be conducted.
- Introductory statement and general investigational plan: the name of the drug and all active ingredients, the drug's structural formula and pharmacologic class, the formulation of dosage form and route of administration, and the broad objectives and planned duration of the study.
- Description of the investigational plan: the rationale for the drug or research study, the indication (s) to be studied, the approach to evaluating the drug, the types of the studies to be conducted, the estimated number of subjects to be given the drug, and any serious risks anticipated based on animal studies or other human experiences with the drug.

- Brief summary of previous human experience with the drug (domestic or foreign), including the reasons if the drug has been withdrawn from any other investigation and/or marketing.
- Chemistry, manufacturing and control information: a complete description of the drug substance including its physical, chemical and biologic characteristics; its method of preparation and analytical methods to ensure its identity, strength, quality, purity, and stability; a quantitative list of the active and inactive components of the dosage form to be administered; the methods, facilities and controls employed in the manufacture, processing, packaging and labelling of the new drug to ensure appropriate qualitative and quantitative standards and product stability during the initial investigation.
- Pharmacologic and toxicology information: the drug's mechanism of action if known; information on drug's absorption, distribution, metabolism, and excretion; and acute, subacute, chronic, reproductive and developmental toxicity studies.
- If the new drug is a combination of previously investigated components, a complete preclinical and clinical summary of these components when administered singly and any data or expectations relating to the effect when combined.
- Clinical protocol of each planned study.
- Commitment that an Institutional Review Board (IRB) has approved the clinical study and will continue to review and monitor the investigation.
- Investigator Brochure.
- Commitment not to begin clinical investigations until the IND is approved, signature of the sponsor or authorised representative, and the date of signed application.

## Clinical Testing (Human Testing, also Known as Clinical Trial)

On successful completion of the pre-clinical testing of the potential molecule, the clinical testing can be initiated after obtaining the regulatory approval based on the Investigational New Drug (IND) application. The testing results of animal model cannot be translated to human beings. Hence, clinical trials are must.

The clinical trial must comply with the ethical and legal requirements of the country. It requires that all studies be approved by the Institutional

Review Board (IRB)/ Institutional Ethics Committee (IEC) at the institutions where trials will take place.

This clinical development phase has four distinct phases:

(i) Phase – I (Initial Human Testing in a small group of healthy volunteers): This phase of trial is performed usually on a small group of healthy human volunteers 20 – 100 in number primarily for the purpose of assuring safety. In some cases, the patients may also be used.

The initial dose of the drug is usually low (one-tenth of the highest no effect dose observed during animal studies). If the first dose is well tolerated, the investigation continues with the administration of progressively greater doses to new subjects until some evidence of the drug's effects are observed.

The pharmacokinetics (absorption, metabolism and elimination) and pharmacodynamics (side effects) are also observed. This helps in determining the safe dosing range.

***The First Dose (Phase I Study):*** The first dose size to be determined, basically depends on three important points:

1. *Safety:* The dose should be as low as possible in order to avoid exposure of the humans to undue risk.

2. *Analytical Sensitivity:* The dose must be high enough to have measurable drug concentration in blood.

3. *Pharmacokinetics:* The dose should be high enough to have drug concentration – time curve in blood measured for at least three times of biological half life, or 10 times of peak concentration.

The first dose can be estimated from $LD_{50}$ values from acute toxicity studies in various species carried out earlier.

Dose should be less than $\dfrac{LD_{50}}{200}$, where $LD_{50}$ is the lowest in any of the tested animal species. For toxic compound the dose should be less than $\dfrac{LD_{50}}{600}$.

(ii) Phase – II (Test in a small group of patients): The Phase II is a controlled clinical study in about 100 – 500 patients with disease to assess the drug's effectiveness, side effects and risks

The phase – II may be divided into Phase IIa and IIb. Phase IIa is a Pilot clinical trial to evaluate efficacy (and safety) in selected populations of patients with the disease or condition to be treated. Phase IIb is a well-controlled trial to evaluate efficacy (and safety) in patients with the disease or condition to be treated. These clinical trials usually represent the most rigorous demonstration of a medicine's efficacy. Sometimes referred to as pivotal trials.

Each patient is monitored for the appearance of the drug's effects while the dose is carefully raised to determine the minimal effective dose. Then the dose is extended beyond the minimum effective dose to the level at which the patient reveals extremely undesirable or intolerable toxic or adverse effects. The greater the range between the minimum effective dose and the dose required to produce severe side effects, the greater is the drug's safety margin.

The phase II studies decide the dose or dose ranges to be used in phase III study.

(iii) Phase – III (Test in a large group of patients to show safety and efficacy): The phase III is a controlled and uncontrolled clinical trial involving around 1000-5000 patients to generate statistically significant data about safety, efficacy and overall benefit-risk relationship of the test drug. Several dosage strengths of the test drug may be evaluated during this phase of study.

The study results provide the basis for labelling instructions to help ensure proper use of the drug including information on potential interactions with other medicines.

Certain phase III studies are continued even after submitting an NDA (with US FDA) but prior to approval to generate additional information: that may support certain labelling requests, provide information on patient's quality of life issues, reveal product advantages over already marketed (reference) drug, provide evidence in support of possible additional drug indications or provide other clues for prospective post - marketing surveillance.

***New Drug Application (NDA):*** On completion of all three phases of study, New Drug Application (NDA) can be filed with Drug Regulatory Authority for seeking marketing approval. The approval is issued on reviewing all data.

***US FDA Requirements (New Drug Application):*** A NDA contains a voluminous data containing both preclinical and clinical results. The preapproval inspection to assess the sponsor's capability to comply with all control and quality standards including GMP is a prerequisite. The applicant has to submit three copies of NDA. The application should contain the following:

- Application form with name, address, date and signature of the applicant or the applicant's authorized representative.

- Chemical, non-proprietary, code, and proprietary names of the drug, the dosage form, its strength and route of administration.

- Statement regarding the applicant's proposal to market the drug product as prescription only or as an OTC product.

- Detailed summary of all aspects of the application, including the proposed text of the product's intended labelling, chemistry, manufacturing and controls, nonclinical and clinical pharmacology and toxicology, human pharmacokinetics and bioavailability, statistical analysis, clinical trial data, benefit and risk considerations, and proposed additional or planned post-marketing studies.

- Detailed technical sections on the chemistry, manufacturing, and controls for the drug substance including its physical and chemical characteristics, method of identification, assay and controls, and the drug product, including its composition, specifications, methods of manufacture and equipments used, in – process controls, batch and master production records, container and closure systems, stability and expiration dating.

- Detailed technical sections for nonclinical pharmacology and toxicology in relation to the proposed therapeutic indication including acute, subacute, and chronic toxicology, carcinogenicity, reproductive toxicology, and animal studies of absorption, distribution, metabolism, and excretion.

- Detailed technical sections of human pharmacokinetics and bioavailability along with microbiology for antibiotic applications.

- Detailed clinical sections for clinical data for each controlled study relating to the proposed indication, a copy of the study protocol, effectiveness and safety data including any updates on safety information, comparison of human and animal pharmacology and toxicology data, support for the dosage and dose intervals and modifications for specific subgroups: paediatric, geriatric, and renal impaired patients.

- Statement regarding compliance to IRB and informed consent requirements.

- Statistical methods and analysis of clinical data.

- Samples of drug substance, drug product proposed for marketing, reference standards, and finished market package, as requested.

- Clinical case report forms for archival copy of the application.

(iv) Phase – IV (Post Marketing Surveillance): Even after the regulatory approval of new drug marketing, the clinical study is continued as a much larger number of patients begin to use the drug. The sponsor/the marketing company needs to continue monitoring the use of drugs carefully and submit periodic reports including the case of adverse effects to the regulatory authority. Such monitoring or reports may help limiting the use of the drug to particular patient groups, or even withdrawal of drug.

*Note:* **Phase – 0** trial also known as microdosing is recently introduced by USFDA that allows researchers to test a small drug dose in fewer human volunteers to quickly weed out drug candidates that are metabolically or biologically ineffective. It includes the administration of single sub-therapeutic dose (generally 1% of pharmacological dose) of a prospective drug to a small number of subjects (10 – 15) to gather preliminary data on drug's pharmacokinetics and pharmacodynamics. A phase 0 study gives no data on safety or efficacy, but carried out to decide which has the best pharmacokinetic parameters in humans to take forward into further development.

## Dosage Forms/Pharmaceutical Products in Clinical Trials

The initial product development is based on the pre-formulation studies and the requirement of dose(s), dosage form, and route of administration desired for clinical trial.

The product usually used in Phase – I and Phase – II may not be very sophisticated or elegant as the final product but must be of high quality and should meet analytical specifications for composition, manufacturing and control and be sufficiently stable for the period of use.

For orally administered drugs, capsules containing pure drug alone without any excipients may be used during Phase – I study. Excipients are included for Phase II trials. During Phase - II, final dosage form is selected out of the several forms tried. For oral administration, blister package is preferred. The final form selected during phase II is used in Phase – III study. This is the formulation (dosage form/ drug product) usually submitted to FDA (US) for seeking marketing approval (NDA).

The dosage form of the test drug and the placebo (or, other reference product) used in controlled clinical trials should be in indistinguishable forms like look alike, taste alike etc. and packaged with coded labels. They need to be manufactured using Good Manufacturing Practice (GMP) facilities.

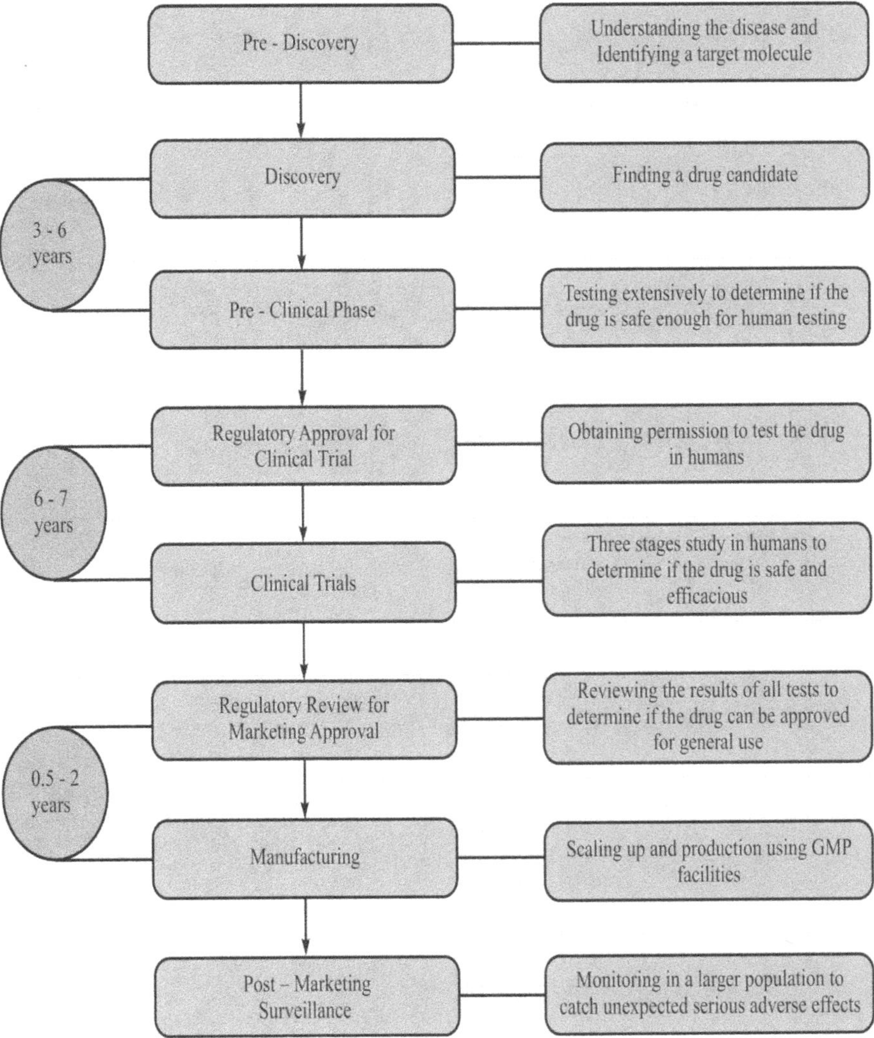


**Fig. 3.1** Sequence of Events in Drug Development.

## Flow Chart of Clinical Trial Approval Process in India

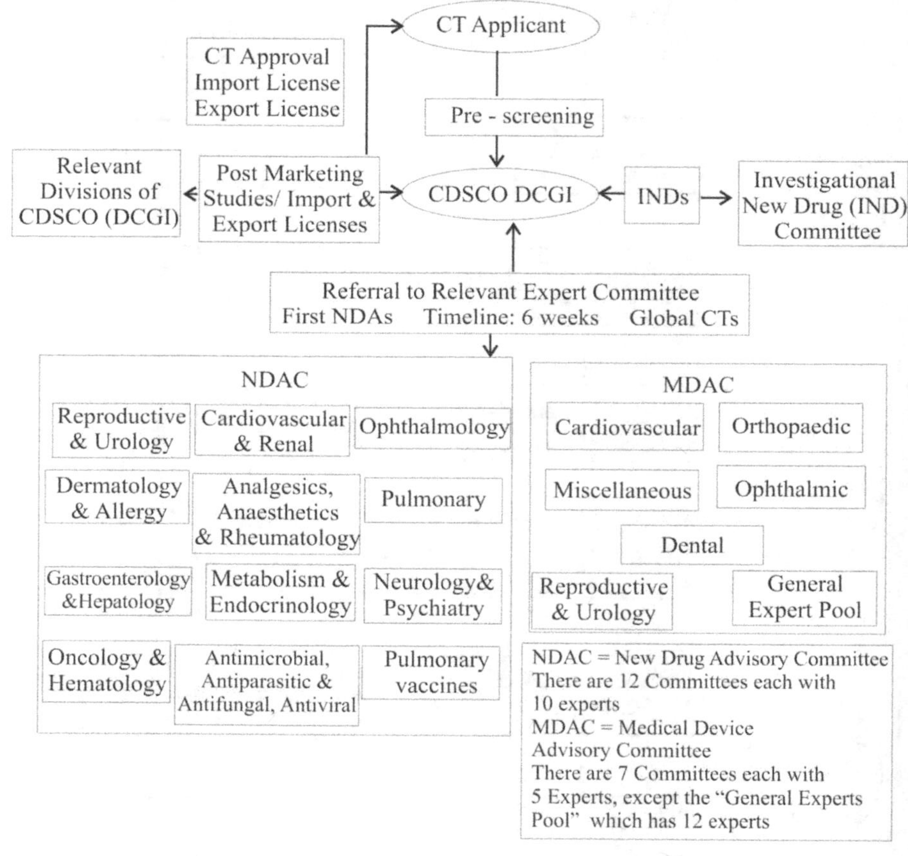

## Key Points to Remember

- Drug discovery is a continuing process. This is of great importance not only for research based pharmaceutical industries but also to meet the healthcare needs of the people. The drug discovery takes about 10-15 years and costing on an average USD 2.6 billion (2014).

- Previously the drugs were discovered through identifying and isolating the active principles from medicinal plants or traditional remedies, or serendipity. But now more rational approach including computer aided drug design is adopted.

- There are six basic approaches used to discover new drugs: identification of new drug target; drug designing based on biological mechanisms, drug receptor structure including CADD; chemical modification of known drug; screening of known products; biotechnology and cloning; and combination of known drugs.

- The promising compound identified is first evaluated in a nimals and this phase is called pre-clinical testing. The animal testing is done to generate all the data that satisfy the safety and efficacy requirements before the new compound is recognized fit to be tested for the first time in humans.

- The animal testing is divided into two broad categories: pharmacological testing and toxicological testing. The pharmacological study includes molecular level study, cellular level study, and whole animal study. The toxicological evaluation covers acute toxicity, sub-acute toxicity, chronic toxicity, reproduction study, carcinogenicity and geno-toxicity. This requirement is specified in Appendix III and IV of Schedule Y.

- The following chemical and pharmaceutical information are required to be submitted to the regulatory authority: information on active ingredient, physic-chemical data, analytical data, complete monograph specification, validation, stability data, and formulation data.

- The investigational new drug application is mandatory for seeking permission for clinical trials. The Appendix I of Schedule Y specifies the data required for submission with application.

- The clinical trials can be conducted only after regulatory and ethics clearance. The clinical trial has four phases and each phase requires approval.

- o The first phase is about initial human testing in small group of healthy volunteers ranging from 20 to 100. The first dose is usually one-tenth of highest no effect dose observed during animal studies.
- o The second phase is a controlled study in about 100-500 patients with disease to assess the drug's effectiveness, side effects and risks. This study decides the dose or dose ranges to be used in next phase.
- o The third phase study is conducted in around 1000-5000 patients to generate statistically significant data on safety and efficacy.
- o The fourth phase is carried out after the drug is approved for study.
- Based on the three phase data, the new drug application can be filed for obtaining marketing approval.

# CHAPTER 4

# Clinical Trials

"Clinical trials are a crucial and necessary aspect of medical research but the highest standards of ethics should be applied at all times, in all countries".

Jessica Sallabank, British Journalist

**After reading this chapter, you should be able to know or learn:**

- The concept and necessity of clinical trials in drug development process;
- Study designs followed in clinical trials;
- Indian regulation to carry out clinical trials;
- Compensation to be paid to trial subjects; and
- Need and methods in Post Marketing Surveillance.

The clinical trial is defined as any investigation in human subjects intended to:

- Discover or verify the clinical, pharmacological and/or other pharmacodynamic effects of an investigational product(s);
- Identify any adverse reactions to an investigational product(s);
- Study absorption, distribution, metabolism and excretion of an investigational product(s)

with an objective of ascertaining its safety and/or efficacy. The term clinical trial is synonymous with clinical study.

In this chapter, the various aspects of clinical trials especially in Indian context are discussed in the following sections.

## Study Design

***Clinical Trial Designs:*** The clinical trials must be well designed to provide highest level of confidence in the validity of the results. Phase – II and some Phase – III studies respectively are controlled. The most important design techniques for avoiding bias in clinical trials are blinding and randomization. Three corner stones of clinical trials are: controls, randomization and blinding. Use of controls, randomization and blinding is the optimum way to ensure that the results are not influenced in a non-random way by external factors. The overall objective in designing a clinical trial is to be able to provide the best possible and most reliable estimate of safety and / or efficacy of the investigational drug.

***Control:*** The controlled trial means the effects of the test drug is compared with either a placebo (placebo control) or a standard drug product (positive control). The placebo control and positive control may be used in the same study. The placebo controlled studies are not encouraged if a standard treatment is available.

The concept of controlled clinical trials is credited to the Frederick II, Roman Emperor who lived from 1192 to 1250 AD. He wanted to know the effect of exercise on digestion. He took two knights for his experiment giving them identical meals. He sent one knight for hunting while to other he asked to sleep. At the end of several hours, he killed both of them and examined the contents of their alimentary canal.

***Blinding*** (Masking) is used to limit the occurrence of conscious and unconscious bias in the conduct and interpretation of a clinical trial. The essential aim is to prevent identification of the treatments until all such opportunities for bias have passed. In a single – blind study the investigator and/or his staff are aware of the treatment but the subjects are kept in dark. On the other hand, a double - blind study means neither the researchers (investigators/sponsor/monitor) nor the subjects know which treatment is delivered until the study is over. The double-blind trial is preferred. This requires that the test product and the placebo or standard reference product should be indistinguishable in terms of appearance, taste etc. either before or during administration.

When double-blinding design is difficult in situations like treatments are different in nature (one surgery and the other drug therapy), two drugs have different formulations, the daily pattern of administration of two treatments may differ; one way of achieving double blind condition is to use double dummy techniques. In double dummy technique, supplies are prepared for treatment A (active and placebo) and for treatment B (active and placebo). The subjects then take two sets of treatment: either A (active) and B (placebo); or A (placebo) and B (active).

Blinding should be broken (decoded) only when it requires during analysis of results or when the knowledge of the treatment assigned is essential for subject's care.

*Randomization* introduces a deliberate element of chance into the assignment of treatments to subjects in a clinical trial. There is random allocation of treatment to subjects. Each subject is assigned randomly to one of the treatments. Different designs require different procedures for generating randomization schedules. In multi centre trials the randomization procedure should be centrally organized. It is preferable to have a random scheme for each centre. Several techniques of randomization: centralized (e.g. allocation by a central office unaware of subject characteristics), pharmacy-controlled randomization, pre-numbered or coded identical containers which are administered serially to participants, on-site computer system combined with allocations kept in a locked unreadable computer file, sequentially numbered, sealed, opaque envelopes.

The **bias in a clinical trial** may be of:
1. *Selection bias*: differences in comparison groups.
2. *Performance bias*: differences in the care provided apart from the intervention being evaluated.
3. *Exclusion bias*: differences in withdrawal from trial.
4. *Detection bias*: differences in outcome assessment.

Three common types of study designs applicable for clinical trials are briefed below:
1. *Parallel Group Design:* The Parallel Group Design may be used for confirmatory trials in which subjects are randomized to one of two or more arms, each arm being allocated a different treatment.

These treatments include the test product at one or more doses, and one or more control treatments (placebo and /or standard reference product).

2. ***Cross Over Design:*** In this type of design, each subject is randomized to a sequence of two or more treatments. Each subject acts as his/her own control for treatment comparison. This reduces the number of subjects and usually the number of assessments.

   In the simplest $2 \times 2$ cross over design, each subject receives each of two treatments in randomized order in two successive treatment periods, separated by a wash out period. The chief concern in cross over study carry over is the residual influence of treatment in subsequent treatment period. The wash out period should be sufficiently long for complete reversibility of drug effect.

3. ***Factorial Design:*** In this type of design, two or more treatments are evaluated simultaneously through the use of varying combinations of the treatments. The simplest example is $2 \times 2$ factorial design in which subjects are randomly allocated to one of the four possible combinations of two treatments. Taking example of two treatments: treatment A and treatment B, the four options are: A alone; B alone; Both A and B, Neither A or B. This type of design is used for specific purpose of examining the interaction of A and B (if treatments are likely to be used together).

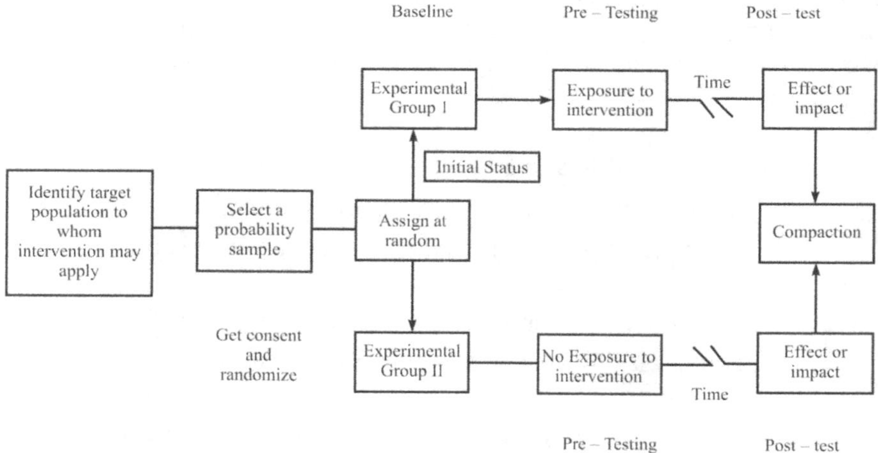


**Fig. 4.1** A typical Design of a Randomized, Controlled, Double Blind Clinical Trial.

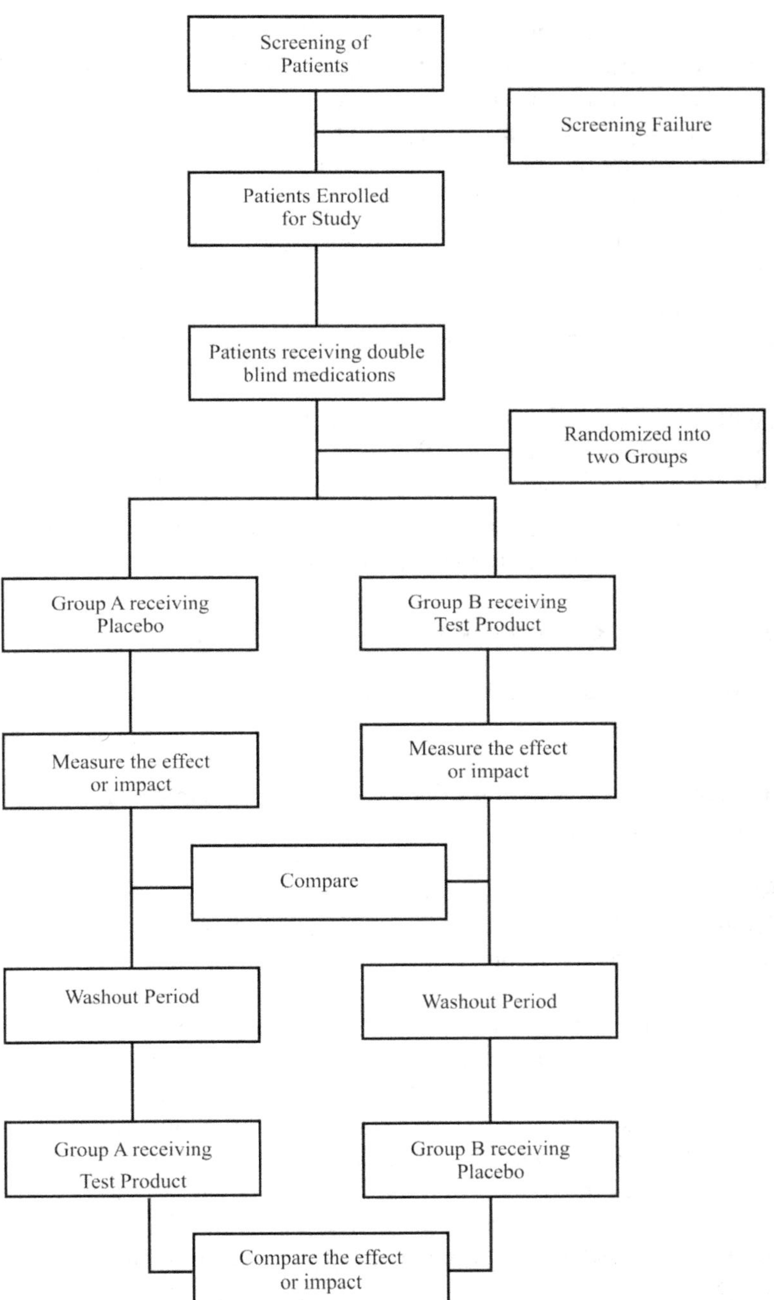



**Fig. 4.2** Randomized Controlled Double Blind Cross Over Design.

**Clinical Trials Outcome:** Efficacy, safety and quality of life are the most accepted indicators used in measuring the outcome of the test drug. Efficacy is an estimate of how effective the investigational or test product is, in eliminating or reducing the symptoms or long term end points of the conditions. Examples of indicators are blood pressure, blood glucose level, tumour size and body mass index.

Safety evaluation includes documentation of all negative adverse effects or events that the trial subjects experience. The investigators monitor these reactions to determine the safety. The adverse events or effects may range from mild like headache to serious such as stroke and death.

Quality of life evaluation involves measurement of physical, mental and social wellbeing, not just the absence of disease or illness. The questionnaires may be on general wellbeing or disease specific.

Trials participants are usually assessed at a minimum of three different time points: Screening, Baseline and End of the trial.

## Regulatory Requirements of Clinical Trials

'The Best Way to Get a Bad Law Repealed is to Enforce it Strictly'

**Abraham Lincoln**

The clinical trial is the testing of new drug(s) in human beings to generate safety and efficacy data required for registration of drug(s). The clinical trial in India is regulated under the Drugs and Cosmetics Act 1940 and the Rules 1945. The main rule that governs the clinical trial is Schedule Y. Though the Schedule Y is first introduced in 1988, it has been amended in 2005 synchronizing the global ethical and Good Clinical Research Practice (GCP). After the exposure of exploitation of study subjects in clinical trials, the government was forced to bring several measures to protect the interest of the trial participants and promoting quality in trial system. In 2013, the Drugs and Cosmetics Rules were amended to make the mandatory registration of ethics committee and provision of compensation payment. The Drugs Controller General (India) (DCGI) is the Licensing Authority under the Act for permitting clinical trials in India. Under the revised Schedule Y the rights of the research participants are protected legalizing the Indian GCP and ethical guidelines.

In this chapter, in addition to salient points of Schedule Y, other regulations like stocking of drugs, conditions for manufacture of drugs for testing, conditions for import of drugs for testing, clinical trial registration are discussed. The readers are encouraged to refer the full text of Schedule Y given in Appendix for further details.

The government has incorporated provisions for payment of compensation in case of injury or deaths during clinical trials. The registration of ethics committee is made mandatory. The government proposes for accreditation system for promoting quality in clinical trial system. The draft rules cover registration of Contract Research Organizations (CROs) mandating strict adherence of standard operating procedures by the individuals, institutions or organizations conducting clinical trials in the country. The CDSCO has also issued separate guidelines 'Guidance for Industry' comprising: Submission of clinical trial application for evaluating safety and efficacy; Requirements for Permission of new drugs approval; Post approval changes in biological products: Quality, Safety and Efficacy Documents; Preparation of quality information for drug information for new drug approval: Biotechnological/Biological products.

**Regulatory Milestones for Clinical Trial**

| | | |
|---|---|---|
| 1952 | – | New drug definition introduced |
| 1970 | – | Guidelines on introduction of new drugs and clinical trials introduced |
| 1988 | – | Schedule Y is introduced (Rules 122 A, B, C – dealing with import or manufacture of new drug for clinical trials) |
| 2001 | – | Rule 122 is amended (Fee Structure etc.) |
| 2001 | – | Post Marketing Surveillance |
| 2001 | – | Indian GCP is introduced |
| 2005 | – | Schedule Y is revised |
| 2009 | – | Mandatory Registration of Clinical Trial |
| 2013 | – | Schedule Y revised incorporating the provision for compensation in case of injury or death (Appendix XII); |
| | - | Mandatory registration of ethics committee |
| | - | Informed consent format is revised incorporating the provision of financial compensation and medical management. |

**Four important terminologies are:** New Drug, Investigational New Drug, Clinical Trial, and Serious Adverse Event.

***New Drug:*** The new drug means: A drug (including bulk drug) which has not been used to any significant extent and has not been recognized as effective and safe for the proposed claims;

An approved drug is now proposed to be marketed with modified or new claims: indications, dosage, dosage forms including sustained release form and route of administration;

A fixed dose combination of two or more drugs, individually approved earlier for certain claims, which are now proposed to be combined for the first time in a fixed ratio. If the ratio is already approved and now proposed to be changed for certain claims is also treated as new drug;

All vaccines are treated as new drugs unless certified otherwise;

A new drug is continued to be considered as new drug for a period of four years from the date of first approval or its inclusion in Indian Pharmacopoeia, whichever is earlier.

***Investigational New Drug:*** A new chemical entity or a product having therapeutic indication but which has never been earlier tested on human beings.

***Clinical Trial:*** A systematic study of new drug(s) in human subject(s) to generate data for discovering and/or verifying the clinical, pharmacological (including pharmacodynamic and pharmacokinetic) and /or adverse effects with the objective of determining safety and/or efficacy of new drug(s).

***Serious Adverse Event:*** A serious adverse event is an untoward medical occurrence during clinical trial that is associated with death, hospitalization, prolongation of hospitalization, persistent or significant disability or incapacity, a congenital anomaly or birth defect or is otherwise life threatening.

***Schedule Y:*** The Schedule Y deals with requirements and guidelines for permission to import and/or manufacture of new drugs for sale or to undertake clinical trial.

***Application for Permission:*** The application for permission to import or manufacture new drugs for sale or to undertake clinical trials is to be made with the following data:

- Chemical and pharmaceutical information
- Animal pharmacology
- Animal toxicology

- Human Clinical Pharmacology:
  - New drugs discovered in India – Trials are required to be carried out right from Phase – I.
  - New drugs discovered in other countries – Phase I data generated outside India is to be submitted. Permission may be granted either to repeat phase – I or to conduct phase – II. Phase III trials are required to be conducted in India prior to marketing approval.
  - The application form must accompany investigator's brochure, proposed protocol, case record form, study subject's informed consent document(s), investigator's undertaking and Ethics Committee's clearance.
  - Regulatory status in other countries: The changes in regulatory status like withdrawal are also to be informed during the course of marketing.
  - Full prescribing information: It should have the following sections: generic name, composition, dosage forms; indications; dose and method of administration; use in special population such as pregnant women, lactating women, paediatric patients, geriatric patients, etc; contraindications; warnings; precautions; drug interactions; undesirable effects; over dose; pharmacodynamic and pharmacokinetic properties; storage and handling instructions.

- Complete testing protocol for quality testing together with complete impurity profile and release specification. Samples of pure drug as well as finished product are to be submitted if required.

  For drugs indicated in life threatening /serious diseases or diseases of special relevance to the Indian health scenario, the toxicological and clinical data requirements may be abbreviated, deferred or omitted as the licensing authority deem appropriate.

***Approval for Clinical Trial:***

- Clinical trial on a new drug can be initiated only after the permission of Licensing Authority (DCGI) and approval of Ethics Committee.

- All trial investigators should possess appropriate qualification, training and experience. A qualified physician or dentist is usually the investigator. Laboratories used for generating data should be compliant with Good Laboratory Practices (GLP).

- All protocol amendments should be notified to the Licensing Authority in writing along with approval of Ethics Committee. No deviation from protocol is permitted without prior approval of Ethics Committee and Licensing Authority except when it is necessary to eliminate immediate hazards. Administrative and logistic changes in the protocol should be notified to the Licensing Authority within 30 days.
- The clinical trials for academic purpose does not require DCGI approval.

### *Responsibility of Regulatory Authority:*

The Drugs Control General India (DCGI) is the Licensing Authority for approving and giving permission to conduct clinical trials. Its responsibilities are:

- Reviewing and approving clinical trial protocols.
- Ensuring that clinical trials comply with ethical and regulatory principles of the country.
- Ensure the payment of compensation in trial related injury.
- Providing registration to ethics committee.

### *Responsibilities of Sponsor:*

- The sponsor is responsible for implementing and maintaining quality assurance system through compliance with GCP. SOPs should be documented to ensure compliance with GCP.
- The sponsor is required to submit a status report to the Licensing Authority at the prescribed periodicity.
- If study is discontinued prematurely, report consisting of brief description of study, the number of patients exposed, dose and duration of exposure, details of adverse drug reactions and reasons for discontinuation, should be submitted within 3 months.
- The responsibility of the sponsor is to bear the medical management expenditure and financial compensation in case of trial related injury. The compensation is to be paid within 30 days of receiving the order from DCGI. The sponsor has to submit the details of compensation paid.
- Unexpected serious adverse event (SAE) should be communicated to the Licensing Authority and others within 10 days of event.

### *Responsibilities of the Investigator(s):*

- The investigator is responsible for conducting the trials based on protocol and GCP guidelines.
- SOPs for the tasks performed are to be documented.
- Ensure adequate medical care for patients for any adverse events.
- Serious and unexpected adverse events should be reported to the sponsor within 24 hours and to the Ethics Committee within 7 days of occurrence.

### *Informed Consent:*

- A written and freely given consent is necessary from each research participant. The investigator must provide written as well as verbal information in a non-technical and understandable language before taking informed consent. The patient information sheet and the patient consent form should be approved by the respective Ethics Committee and furnished to the Licensing Authority.
- In case of unconscious person or minor or persons suffering from illness or disability where the individual is not in a position to give own written consent, legally acceptable representative may give the consent. If the legally acceptable representative is unable to read or write the whole process should be conducted in presence of an impartial witness.
- Appendix V now contains the additional statement describing the financial compensation and medical management.

**ICH and Informed Consent Form:** The ICH specifies the following 20 issues to be addressed in a layman's language in written form: 1. The trial involves research; 2. Purpose of trial; 3. Trial treatments; 4. Trial procedures; 5. The participant's responsibilities; 6. Experimental trial aspects; 7. Foreseeable risks or inconveniences; 8. Expected benefits; 9. Alternative procedures or treatments; 10. Compensation and / or treatment available in the event of trial related injury; 11. Payment to participant; 12. Expenses for participant; 13. Participation is voluntary and the participant may refuse to participate or withdraw from a trial at any time; 14. The monitors, auditors, EC and the regulatory authorities will be granted direct access to the participant's medical records; 15. Records' identifying the participant will be kept confidential;

16. The participants or representative will be informed if information becomes available that may be relevant to their willingness to continue participating in the trial; 17. Person(s) to contact for further information regarding the trial, rights of trial participants and in the event of trial related injury; 18. Circumstances or the reasons under which the participation may be terminated; 19. Expected duration of trial participation; and 20. Approximate number of participants in the trial.

### *Responsibilities of the Ethics Committee:*

- The EC should take care to safe guard the rights, safety and well being of all research participants especially the vulnerable subjects. It should have the SOPs and maintain a record of its proceedings.

- It must review the trials periodically based on progress report submitted including visiting trial site.

- Revoking the approval decision must be communicated to the investigator and the Licensing Authority.

- Decides the number of clinical trials one investigator can conduct.

- Approves the trial sites.

More details on the role of ethics committee are available in the separate chapter.

### *Human Pharmacology (Phase – I):*

- This is done in healthy human volunteers usually by investigators trained in Clinical Pharmacology to estimate the safety and tolerability. For drugs with potential toxicity like anti-cancer drugs, the study is to be done in patients only. There must be facilities to closely observe and monitor the subjects.

- The study is usually intended with the following objectives:
  - To determine the maximum tolerated dose.
  - To determine pharmacokinetic parameters in different age groups to support dosing recommendations and formulation development.
  - To generate pharmacodynamic data which are helpful in deciding dosage and dosage regimen.
  - To measure preliminary drug activity especially when tested in patients.

### *Therapeutic Exploratory Trials (Phase – II):*

- This is done to evaluate the effectiveness for a particular indication(s) and to determine the common short term side effects and risks. Another objective is to determine the dose and dosage regimen for Phase – III trial. Doses used in phase – II are usually (but not always) less than the highest doses used in Phase – I.

- This is done with another objective in mind-to determine study end points, therapeutic regimens (including concomitant medications) and target population (mild versus severe diseases) for further studies in Phase II and III.

- In case of global study, the details like number of sites and the patients including justification for conducting study in India is to be submitted.

### *Therapeutic Confirmatory Trials (Phase – III):*

- The Phase – III is designed to confirm the preliminary evidence accumulated in Phase – II that a drug is safe and effective for use in the intended indication and recipient population. The study further confirms dose-response relationship, use in wider populations, in different stages of disease, safety and efficacy in combination with other drug(s). The data generated from the adequate basis for getting marketing approval.

- Trials in Phase – III helps generating prescribing information especially for drugs intended for use for a long period.

- For already approved drugs outside India, Phase – III is to be carried out in India to generate evidence of efficacy and safety of drug before approval for marketing. It may also be necessary to do pharmacokinetic studies to verify the data generated in Indian population is in conformity with the data already generated abroad.

- For global trials, the details like number of sites and the patients including justification for conducting study in India is to be submitted.

### *Post Marketing Trials (Phase – IV):*

These are not necessary for new drug approval but are required for optimising the drug use. The Phase –IV trials include additional drug-drug interaction(s), dose – response or safety studies and trials designed to support use under approved indication(s), mortality/morbidity studies, epidemiological studies etc.

**Studies in Special Populations:** If the drug is intended for use in children, pregnant women, nursing women, elderly patients, patients with renal or other organ failures, and on those on specific concomitant medication, it is necessary to submit the relevant data.

*Geriatrics:* Geriatric patients should be included in phase III (and phase II if sponsor decides) in meaningful numbers if:

- the disease intended to be treated is characteristically a disease of aging; or
- the population to be treated is known to include substantial number of geriatric patients; or
- when there are likely that the conditions common to elderly are encountered; or
- the new drug is likely to have different response in elderly compared to non-geriatric patients.

*Paediatric:* If the drug is intended for children, evaluation should be made in the appropriate age group. It is usually appropriate to begin the study with older children before extending the trial to younger children and then infants.

- The initial safety and tolerability data is usually obtained in adults and then the trial in this population.
- If the drug is intended to treat serious or life threatening diseases occurring both in adults and paediatric patients, for which there are currently no or limited therapeutic option, the paediatric population may be included.
- The studies in paediatric population at various phases of clinical development or after post marketing surveillance in adults if safety concerns exists.
- The studies should include: clinical trials, relative bioequivalence of paediatric formulation, paediatric pharmacokinetic.
- If the new drug is a major therapeutic advance, the study should begin early in the drug development process and this data should be submitted with the new drug application.
- Written informed consent should be obtained from the parent/legal guardian. However all paediatric participants should be informed of the study in an understandable language. The mature minors and adolescents should   personally sign and date a separately designed written consent form.

- The reviewing ethics committee should include members knowledgeable about paediatric, ethical, clinical and psychosocial issues.

### Pregnant or Nursing Women

Pregnant or Nursing Women should be included in clinical trials only when the drug is intended for use by pregnant or nursing mother or foetus or nursing infant and where the data generated from non-pregnant/non-nursing women is not suitable.

For drugs intended for use during pregnancy, follow up data on the pregnancy, foetus, and child is required. Where applicable, excretion of the drug or its metabolite into human milk should be examined and the infant should be monitored for possible pharmacological effects.

***Post Marketing Surveillance:*** Post Marketing Surveillance is the safety monitoring of new drugs while they are in use (market). It is necessary to submit Periodic Safety Update Reports (PSUR) in order to:

- Report all relevant new information from appropriate sources;

- Relate these data to patient exposure;

- Summarize the market authorization status in different countries and any significant variations related to safety; and

- Indicate whether changes should be made to product information in order to optimize the use of product.

- The single PSUR should have all dosage forms and indications but with separate presentations.

- The PSURs should be submitted every six months for first two years after approval and then annual submission for next two years. The PSUR should cover only the period of the report (interval). The serious unexpected adverse reaction must be reported to the Licensing Authority within 15 days of initial receipt of information.

- New studies specifically planned or conducted to examine a safety issue should be described in the PSURs.

- Structure of PSUR:
    - ✓ Title page containing periodic safety update report for the product, applicant's name, period covered by the report, date of approval of the new drug, date of marketing of new drug and date of reporting;
    - ✓ Introduction;

- ✓ Current worldwide market authorization status;
- ✓ Update of actions taken for safety reason; changes in safety information;
- ✓ Estimated patient exposure;
- ✓ Presentation of individual case histories;
- ✓ Studies;
- ✓ Other information;
- ✓ Overall safety evaluation;
- ✓ Conclusion; and
- ✓ Appendix providing material relating to indications, dosing, pharmacology and other related information.

### *Special Studies: Bioavailability/Bioequivalence Studies:*

- If the drug is approved outside India and absorbed systemically, bioequivalence study should be carried out wherever applicable. These studies should be conducted under labelled conditions of administration. Data to the extent of absorption may be required for formulation not meant for systemic absorption.

- Effect of food on drug absorption should be studied.

- Data from dissolution studies for all solid dosage forms are required.

- Dissolution and bioavailability data submitted with the new drug application must provide information that assures bioequivalence or establishes bioavailability and dosage correlations between the product intended for marketing and the product used in clinical trial.

- All bioavailability and bioequivalence studies should be conducted according to the guidelines for Bioavailability and Bioequivalence Studies as issued by CDSCO.

  Depending upon the nature of new drug(s) and the disease(s), additional information may be required by the Licensing Authority. The applicant needs to certify the authenticity of submitted data and documents. The Licensing Authority reserves the right to reject any data or any document if they are of doubtful integrity.

### *There are 12 appendices attached to Schedule Y. They are*

- Appendix I: Data to be submitted along with the application to conduct clinical trials/import/manufacture of new drugs for marketing in the country.

- Appendix IA: Data required to be submitted by an applicant for grant of permission to import and/or manufacture a new drug already approved in the country.
- Appendix II: Structure, Contents, and Format for Clinical Study Reports.
- Appendix III: Animal Toxicology (Non-Clinical Toxicity Studies).
- Appendix IV: Animal Pharmacology.
- Appendix V: Informed Consent.
- Appendix VI: Fixed Dose Combinations (FDCs).
- Appendix VII: Undertaking by the Investigator.
- Appendix VIII: Ethics Committee including registration.
- Appendix IX: Stability Testing of New Drugs.
- Appendix X: Contents of the Proposed Protocol for Conducting Clinical Trials.
- Appendix XI: Data elements for reporting serious adverse events occurring in a clinical trial.
- Appendix XII: Compensation in case of injury or death during clinical trial.

## Registration of Clinical Trials

There has been increasing concern over the influence of industry on clinical trials. This is because the pharmaceutical companies can make higher profits if the trial reaches favourable conclusions. Bias created in clinical trials can bring out inaccurate information which is often used as evidence on safety, efficacy and quality of drugs. In order to avoid this allegation and improve better safe guarding the health of the people, a mandatory disclosure of the results from drugs trials is recommended. Such data are expected to be made public within one year of the end of the trials. Registration of clinical trials is necessary even to publish the results in journals.

Taking steps in this direction, the Government of India made the clinical trial registration mandatory. Each and every clinical trial requires to be registered with clinical trial registry managed by Indian Council of Medical Research (ICMR) before initiating a clinical trial with effect from 15th June 2009. Though initially, when the registry was floated, it was optional to register but now it is mandatory. The Clinical Trials Registry- India (CTRI) has been set up by the ICMR's National Institute of Medical Statistics (NIMS) and is funded by the Department of Science and Technology (DST) through the Indian Council of Medical Research (ICMR). It also receives financial and technical support through the WHO, WHO-SEARO, and the WHO India Country office. The official website: www.ctri.in. Registration of trials ensures transparency, accountability and accessibility of clinical trials and their results. Further, it promotes greater trust and public confidence in clinical research. Trial registration also helps to prevent bias generated by selective reporting of only "positive" findings as well as reduce unnecessary duplication of research through greater awareness of existing trials and results.

The CTRI [http://www.ctri.nic.in/Clinicaltrials/login.php] is an online register of clinical trials being conducted in India. Any researcher who plans to conduct a trial involving human participants, of any intervention (drug, surgical procedure, preventive measures, lifestyle modifications, devices, educational or behavioural treatment, rehabilitation strategies and complementary therapies) needs to register the trial in CTRI before enrolment of the first participant.

The "Responsible Registrant" for a trial is either the principal investigator (PI) or the primary sponsor, to be decided by an agreement between the parties. The primary sponsor is ultimately accountable for ensuring that the trial is properly registered. For multi-center and multi-sponsor trials, it is the lead PI or lead sponsor who should take responsibility for registration. However, in case of multi-country trials, the Indian PI should also get the trial registered in CTRI quoting any other Registration number as its Secondary ID.

***The following items are to be recorded (This includes WHO Data Set Items)***

1. Unique Trial Reference Number (UTRN): is given by WHO.
2. Registration Number.
3. Trial Registration date.
4. Public Title of the Study.
5. Scientific Title of the Study (Give Trial Acronym if any).
6. Secondary IDs if any.
7. Principal Investigator's Name and Address.
8. Contact Person (Scientific Query).
9. Contact Person (Public Query).
10. Funding Source(s).

11. Primary Sponsor.
12. Secondary Sponsor.
13. Name of Ethics Committee and Approval Status.
14. Regulatory Clearance obtained from DCGI.
15. Date of first enrolment.
16. Estimated Duration of trial.
17. Target Sample Size.
18. Health Condition/Problem Studied.
19. Intervention and Comparator Agent.
20. Key Inclusion/Exclusion Criteria.
21. Primary Outcome/s.
22. Secondary Outcome/s.
23. Countries of Recruitment.
24. Site(s) of Study.
25. Status of Trial.
26. Phase of Trial.
27. Study Type.
28. Brief Summary.
29. Method of Generating Randomization Sequence.
30. Method of Allocation Concealment.
31. Blinding and Masking.

The procedure for registering a trial is given in the website. Basically it involves creating a login ID and password. Then the necessary information is to be submitted online. On submission of all relevant data, a trial will be registered and allocated a unique registration number. The date of submission and date of registration are recorded.

As the registration of clinical trials are made mandatory, there has been an increasing momentum in number of clinical trial registration. Besides this, the Indian Registry has been receiving application from other countries too. Under this scenario, the Government of India proposes to incorporate numerous other provisions like auditing of trial in the registry in order to make it inline of international standards.

## Conditions of Import of Drugs for Examination, Test or Analysis

- Small quantities of drugs can be imported for the purpose of examination, test or analysis (which is otherwise prohibited) under licence from DCGI (CDSCO).
- A license is usually valid for one year.
- The licensee should use the imported substances for the purpose for which the import licence is issued (exclusively for examination, test or analysis).
- Drugs Inspector should be allowed, with or without prior notice, to inspect the premises where such drugs are kept and investigate the manner of using the drugs including taking samples.
- All records relating to import are to be kept and the details like quantity imported, date of importation and the name of the manufacturer need to be reported to the Licensing Authority.
- Licensee has to comply with additional requirements as subsequently prescribed, within one month's notice.
- A license is necessary for examination, test or analysis for which an application is to be made countersigned by the Head of the institution in which, or by a proprietor or director the company or firm by which the examination, test or analysis will be conducted.
- A license for examination, test or analysis can be cancelled by the Licensing Authority for breach of any condition. An aggrieved person whose license is cancelled can appeal to the Central Government  within three months of date of order of cancellation.

## Conditions for Manufacture of Drugs for Examination, Test or Analysis

- Small quantities of drugs (which are otherwise are most prohibited) can be manufactured under a license for manufacturing from the State Licensing Authority (State Drugs Controller).
- The manufactured drug should be kept in containers bearing labels indicating the purpose for which it has been manufactured (examination, test or analysis).
- If the manufactured drug is supplied to other person, the label on the container should state the name and address of manufacturer,

scientific name (or a reference for identification) and the purpose of its manufacturing.

- If the proposed manufacturer does not hold other manufacturing licences, it is necessary to obtain license for manufacturing drugs for purposes of examination, test or analysis. If such drugs are not recognized as safe for use, a license would not be issued unless the DCGI issues no objection to this effect.

- The license is usually valid for one year which may be renewable for one year at a time. The license can be suspended or cancelled if licensee fails to comply with conditions of license. An aggrieved person may approach the state government within three months of receipt of such order of suspension or cancellation.

- The manufactured drugs should be exclusively used for the purpose of examination, test or analysis. The manufacturing, examination, test or analysis should be carried out at the specified place only.

- Drugs Inspector should be allowed, with or without prior notice, to inspect the premises where drugs are manufactured and to satisfy him/her that only examination, test or analysis work is being conducted.

- Records related to manufacturing and the person(s) to whom the drugs have been supplied.

- Licensee has to comply with additional requirements as subsequently prescribed within one month's notice.

- The licensee has to maintain an Inspection Book to enable drugs inspector to record his impressions and defects noticed.

**Export of Biological Specimens of Clinical Trials:** The biological samples collected during clinical trial process can be exported to other laboratories located outside India for test or analysis under a license from Director General of Foreign Trade, Government of India. However, in order to apply for such license, it is necessary to obtain No Objection Certificate (NOC) from DCGI. The DCGI has proposed the following format for submitting application for obtaining NOC:

Application format to be submitted in the O/o DCG(I) for sending biological Sample of Clinical trial for testing through DGFT

| 1 | **Name and address of the firm** | | |
|---|---|---|---|
| 2. | **Type of Application**<br>(Global Trial/Bioequivalence Study/Others) | | |
| 3. | **Name of the Drug** | | |
| 4. | Purpose of the Export of biological samples whether any permission granted by this Directorate for Clinical Trial of the subject drug.  If so furnish the copy of the same. | | |
| 5. | Tentative date of completion of Clinical Trial | | |
| 6. | Import Export Code Number (I.E.C No.) | | |
| 7. | **Type of Sample** | **IMPORT TARIFF CODE (ITC CODE)** | **Quantity of Samples** |
| | - Whole human Blood e.g<br>Serum<br>Plasma<br>Urine<br>Others | | |
| 8. | - Shipment Details<br>- Port of Loading<br>  Port of Discharge<br>- Country of Export | | |
| 9. | Name and address of the laboratory where analysis to be conducted. | | |
| 10. | Whether application is already submitted in DGFT, if so, submit the copy of the same | | |

**(Signature of the Competent
Authority/Head of the Institute/Firm with date)**

**In a meeting (17th October 2006) of the Drugs Controller General (India), Manufacturer Associations like IDMA, OPPI, IPA, CROs and Individual Specialists in the field of Clinical Trials following decisions (salient Points) were taken:**

1. For the purpose of granting permission, the clinical trials are classified into category A and category B. The category A includes those clinial trials whose protocols are approved by some of the recognised and developed countries like USA, UK, Switzerland, Australia, Canada, Germany, South Africa, Japan, EMEA.  In this cases the permission will be granted accepting the approval of protocols by the countries mentioned above. And the time frame suggested for such clearances based on the current load of 20

applicatons per month is 2 – 4 weeks and the members have agreed that such  time frame will help them to meet the global timelines.

All the other applications which are not covered under category A fall  under category B. They will take more time as the adequacy of the protocol have to be verified to protect the subjects. The approximate time for this is excepted to be  8 – 12 weeks.  It was clarified that once an application is considered under category B it will not be shifted to category A even though the applicant produces an approval from the developed countries mentioned above the protocols.

2.  As a part of the data to be submitted for each phase of clinical trial, it was agreed upon to accept summarized information in investigatiors brochure duly supported by an affidavit declaring that the information furnished in the summarised affidavit are based on the facts.

3.  The summarised information shall include information with respect to safety and efficacy of these drugs.

4.  As regarding Phase I Clinical Trial, DCG(I) has clarified the Government Policy that the Phase I trials are permitted to those molecules which are discovered in India.

5.  He also stated that the repeat Phase I can also be permitted to the company.

6.  As regarding request for permitting Phase I studies on repeat dose limiting to the total dose maximum to single dose, same will be examined in consultation with experts and decison will be taken on the basis of discussions.

7.  As regarding Phase IV trials if the drug is permitted for marketing into India, it will be permitted and will be considered as "Category A" and in case if the drug is not permitted it will be kept under category B for complete examination.

8.  DCG (I) also opinioned to find out and prepare a list in consultation with experts indications for which Phase IV clinical trials should not be permitted.

9.  DCG (I) re-emphasised that incomplete applications are one of the major reasons for delay in clearances and stated that once  the checklist and information to be furnished is finalised, any application not complying with the requirements will stand rejected and no correspendence will be entertained.  The applicant has to re-apply with necessary fees etc., as per rules and he will get his chance based on the receipt of the application second time.

10. As regarding protocol amendments, it was agreed upon after deliberations to categorise the amendments into three categories : a. Those amendments which do not require any information or permission b. Those amendements which require to be infomed but need not wait for permission. c. Those amendments which require prior permission before implementation of the amendments.

11. DCG (I) desired that the CROs carrying out the global clinical trials and should submit half yearly returns on the status of Clinical Trials which were permitted by him as per standard format and communicated through the website.

12. DCG (I) also informed that all permissions granted will be registered and maintained for the purpose by DCG (I)

13. After deliberations it was agreed upon that the CROs while submitting serious adverse events will also provide a proof from the sponsorer to have intimated the respective regulatory bodies with whom they are filing the data.

14. The DCG (I) suggested to simplify the procedure of issuing NOC for test license, clinical trial and export of serum samples in one permission letter as against the current practice of three permission letters. He desired that the time of application for global Clinical Trial should also include applications for test license and if they propose to send any of the samples abroad for test and analysis, those information shall also be given along with the application.

15. As regarding destruction of drugs imported by manufacturer for the purpose of Clinical trials shall be carried out by the CROs / Sponsor and the certificate to the extent shall be furnished along with the returns they are going to file half-yearly.

16. The members present in the meeting desired that audit should be initiated by the investigators and the ethical committees. DCG (I) has agreed to the suggestion and said to workout for the same.

17. DCG (I) also wanted to know the views of the participating members about need for self regulators as well as regulations from the regulatory authorities. All the participating members have expressed their need for regulation of organisation carrying out Clinical Trials by the regulatory mechanism.

The following requirements were finalized for submission of applications for Global Clinical Trials:

## Requirements for Filling Applications for Global Clinical Trial

## (for submission of data to countries other than India )

1. Name of the Applicant
2. Authorization letter from the Sponsor
3. Name of the Drug
4. Regulatory status of the drug in other countries (Names of countries where the drug is approved along with international package insert or where IND application is filed)
5. Objective of the Study
6. Phase of Study
7. Names of the Participating Countries /Investigator sites
8. Total no. of patients to be enrolled globally
9. No. of investigator sites to be enrolled in India
10. No. of patients to be included in India
11. Regulatory/ IRB approvals from participating countries

    (these approvals should be submitted along with their English translation and reason incase the company is submitting an expired IRB/ IEC approval)
12. Status of the study in other countries

    (this should include no. of patients enrolled, no. of patients completed the study and no. of patients discontinued)
13. Suspected Unexpected Serious Adverse Reaction (SUSAR) from other participating countries if any reported
14. Affidavit from the sponsor that the study has not been discontinued in any country and in case of discontinuation the reasons for such a discontinuation and that the applicant would further communicate to DCG (I) about future discontinuation
15. Data Submitted
    (a) Chemical and Pharmaceutical data
        (i) Generic name and chemical name
        (ii) Dosage form
        (iii) Composition
    (b) Animal Pharmacology Data
    (c) Animal Toxicology data
    (d) Clinical data
        (i) Phase I          (ii) Phase II
        (iii) Phase III       (iv) Phase IV
    (e) Rationale for selecting the proposed dose(s) and indication(s)
16. Documents Submitted
    (a) Form 44 (Drugs and Cosmetics Act and the Rules) and Treasury chalan
    (b) Form 12 (Drugs and Cosmetics Act and the Rules) and Treasury chalan

(c) Details of Biological specimens to be exported

(d) Protocol

(e) Informed Consent Documents (ICD)

(f) Case Report form

(g) Investigator's Brochure duly supported by an affidavit that the summarized information submitted is based on facts

(h) Undertakings by the Investigators

(i) Ethics committee approvals (if already available)

## Protocol Amendments

(a) Those amendments which do not require notification or permission of the Licensing Authority

   (i) Administrative and Logistic changes

   (ii) Minor protocol amendments and additional safety assessments incase the institutional ethics committee has already approved these changes

(b) Those amendments which require notification to the Licensing Authority but need not wait for permission

   (i) Additional Investigator sites

   (ii) Change in investigator with the consent to withdraw from the earlier investigator

   (iii) Amended Investigators Brochure, amended informed consent form

(c) Those amendments which require prior permission of the Licensing Authority

   (i) Additional Patients to be recruited

   (ii) Major changes in protocol with respect to study design, dose and treatment options

   (iii) Any change in inclusion or exclusion criteria

**Note:** All amendments must be approved by the concerned Institutional Ethics Committee before their implementation

(Source CDSCO website: accessed on 15th January 2010)

### Compensation incase of injury or death during clinical trial

This provision is introduced with an amendment of Drugs and Cosmetics (First Amendment) Rules, 2013. The salient points and the formula for fixing the quantum of compensation are given below.

1. In case of injury, the clinical trial subject(s) should be given free medical treatment as long as required;

2. If injury is related to clinical trial, the subject(s) are entitled for financial compensation as ordered by the DCGI, the Licensing Authority. The financial compensation is over and above any expenses incurred on the medical management of the subject;

3. In case of trial related death, the nominee of the deceased is entitled for financial compensation which is over and above the expenses incurred on medical management;

4. The sponsor of the trial is responsible for paying the medical management expenses and bear the financial compensation as well;

5. Clinical trial injury or death if due to the following reasons, then the trial subject or the nominee is entitled for financial compensation:

    (a) Adverse effects of investigational product(s);

    (b) Violation of the approved protocol, scientific misconduct or negligence by the sponsor or his representative or the investigator;

    (c) Failure of the investigational product to provide intended therapeutic effect;

    (d) Use of placebo in a placebo controlled study;

    (e) Adverse effects due to concomitant medication excluding standard care, necessitated as a part of approved protocol;

    (f) For injury to a child *in–utero* because of participation of parent in clinical trial; and

    (g) Any clinical trial procedures involved in the study.

6. Sponsor is required to give an undertaking along with the application for clinical trial submission to the licensing authority to provide compensation;

7. The Licensing Authority constitutes independent expert committee to decide on the reason of injury and the quantum of compensation. The guideline on deciding the quantum of compensation is described later in the chapter.

8. The sponsor is required to submit the details of compensation provided or paid for clinical trial related injury or death to the Licensing Authority within 30 days of receiving order from the Licensing Authority.

9. If the sponsor fails to provide medical management or financial compensation, the licensing authority may suspend or cancel the clinical trial and/or restrict the sponsor or his representative to conduct any further trial in the country. The procedure of show cause notice is to be followed;

10. Responsibilities of different stake holders:

| Stake holders | Injury other than death | Death |
| --- | --- | --- |
| Sponsor | After due analysis the sponsor has to report to the chairman of ethics committee, Licensing Authority and Head of the Institution of trial site within 10 calendar days of the event. | 1. The sponsor has to report the event to the Head of the Institution of trial site at the earliest.<br>2. After due analysis, the sponsor has to report to the chairman of ethics committee, chairman of expert committee with a copy of report to the Licensing Authority, and Head of the Institution of the trial site within 10 calendar days of the event. |
| Investigator | The investigator has to report all serious and unexpected adverse events to the Licensing Authority, the sponsor or his representative, and ethics committee within 24 hours of their occurrence. | The investigator, after due analysis, has to forward its report to the chairman of EC, chairman of expert committee with a copy to Licensing Authority and Head of the Institution of the trial site within 10 calendar days of the event. |
| Ethics Committee | After due analysis and giving opinion on financial compensation if any, EC has to report the Licensing Authority within 21 calendar days of the event. | After due analysis along with the opinion on financial compensation , the EC has to submit the report to expert committee with a copy of the report to the Licensing Authority within 21 calendar days of the event. |

*Contd...*

| Stake holders | Injury other than death | Death |
|---|---|---|
| Independent Expert Committee [formed by Licensing Authority] | The committee has to find out the cause of event and decides on the quantum of compensation [No direct reporting of EC to expert committee] | 1. The committee has to find out the cause of event and quantum of compensation.<br>2. To report to the Licensing Authority within 30 calendar days of receiving the report of EC. |
| Licensing Authority | The Licensing Authority has to:<br>1. Find out the cause of event and quantum of compensation [may be from an independent expert committee].<br>2. Pass the order within three months of receiving report of the event. | The Licensing Authority has to:<br>1. Find out the cause of event and quantum of compensation from an independent expert committee.<br>2. Pass the order within three months of receiving report of the event. |

**Compensation Formula:** The DCGI constituted three independent expert committees on 14th March 2013 under the chairmanship of Dr. A. K. Agarwal of Maulana Azad Medical College, New Delhi, to examine the Serious Adverse Events of deaths occurring during clinical trials and to recommend the cause of death, and to determine the quantum of compensation. The committee after due deliberation finally adopted the following principles:

1. The criteria should not be discriminative in nature: no discrimination on socio-economic conditions – education, income etc.;

2. The criteria should not discriminate gender;

3. The criteria should not be such, which may have minimal impact but may create large variability;

4. The formula should be such that the inter-group variability of compensation value so arrived at has little scope of discretion, thus avoids possible bias;

5. The criteria should include age of the subject as one of the factors; and

6. The criteria should consider risk factors in the formula depending on the seriousness and severity of the disease, presence of comorbidity and duration of disease of the subject at the time of enrolment in the clinical trial.

Three following factors are used in calculation for deriving the compensation amount:

(a) Age of the subject: This is adopted from Workmen Compensation Act. The factor ranges from 99.37 (for age of 65 or more) to 228.54 (of age not more than 16). More details are given in Appendix.

(b) Risk factors: The risk factor is divided into five grade scale of 0.50, 1.0, 2.0, 3.0 and 4.0 in case of patients whose expected mortality is 90% or more within 30 days, the fixed amount of Rs. 2 lakh may be given. The five grades are:

 1. 0.50 [Terminally ill patient with expected survival of not more than 6 months];
 2. 1.0 [patient with high risks and expected survival between 6 to 24 months];
 3. 2.0 [Patient with moderate risks];
 4. 3.0 [Patient with mild risk]; and
 5. 4.0 [Healthy volunteers or subject with no risks].

(c) Base Amount: The base amount should be such that if the nominee of the subjects keeps that amount of compensation in bank by way of fixed deposit, the he / she will get a monthly interest amount which is at least approximately equivalent to the minimum wages of the unskilled workers. The base amount is decided to be Rs. 8.0 lakh referring to the age of 65 years (corresponding factor of 99.37).

$$\text{Compensation} = \frac{B \times F \times R}{99.37}$$

Where B = Base amount (8 Lakh),

       F = Factor depending upon the age of the subject,

       R = Risk factors depending upon the seriousness and severity of the disease.

***The above formula is for SAE causing deaths.***

(d) In case of patients whose expected mortality is 90% or more within 30 days, a fixed amount of Rs. 2 lakh should be given.

The minimum amount specified is Rs. 2 lakh and the maximum amount is Rs. 73.60 lakh.

(e) The formula specified above is provisional one. The committee will examine the cases of serious adverse events of deaths and decides the final quantum of compensation after due diligence and application of mind on the risk factor and recommend the same to DCGI on case to case basis.

**Compensation for trial related injury other than deaths:** The following categories of injuries are entitled for compensation:

(a) A permanent disability,

(b) Congenital anomaly or birth defects,

(c) Chronic life threatening disease, or

(d) Reversible serious adverse event in case it is resolved.

**Compensation formula for permanent disability** $= \dfrac{(C \times D \times 90)}{100 \times 100}$

Where

D = Percentage disability the subject has suffered

C = Quantum of compensation which would have been due for payment to the subject(s) in case of death

**Serious Adverse Events causing congenital anomaly or birth defect** may have:

(i) Still birth

(ii) Early death due to anomaly

(iii) No death but deformity which can be fully corrected through appropriate intervention

(iv) Permanent disability (mental or physical)

**The quantum of compensation is equal to half of the amount as derived for death. In case of III and IV types, the medical management is to be provided over above financial compensation.**

**Compensation for chronic life threatening disease or reversible SAE in case it is resolved:**

Compensation $= 2 \times W \times N$

Where W = Minimum wage per day of the unskilled worker

N = Number of days of hospitalization

## Post Marketing Surveillance (PMS)

The new drugs have undergone a significant amount of testing and evaluation through animal testing and clinical trials before being receiving marketing authorization. This is done to ensure that the product is of good quality, effective, and safe. While the quality and effectiveness can be assessed with certainty, the issue of safety is less certain. There are no drugs that are free of side effects or adverse drug reactions though incidence may vary.

The clinical trials are incomplete studies with regard to drug safety (to possible ADRs) due to several reasons:

- Animal testing data cannot be completely used to predict the safety in humans.

- Selected and limited numbers of patients are used in clinical trials, while a large number of patients get exposure to the drug during actual clinical practice.

- The duration of trial is limited.

- Information about rare and serious adverse drug reactions, chronic toxicity, and use in special groups like children, elderly or pregnant women or drug interaction is incomplete or not generated.

The clinical trials can uncover the commonest Adverse Drug Reactions (ADRs) (>1% incidence). Less common ADRs (<1%) can be discovered only on long term study in large population. A study of 500 subjects is required to detect a risk occurring once in 100 research participants and a study of 3000 research participants are needed to detect a 1: 1000 risks. This implies the need of continuing the process of evaluating the drug safety in the post approval period. This post approval phase of safety study is known as post marketing surveillance. The post marketing surveillance is defined as scientific study of a product that is approved for marketing, designed to produce reliable information about the drug safety. Though PMS is included as part of clinical trial (phase – IV), it is not appropriate.

Although the PMS involves the study of both the efficacy (new indications or actual benefits) and safety after marketing approval, the term has most generally linked to long term assessment of adverse effects of drug use. The PMS is carried out using the Pharmacovigilance programme prevailing in the country. Pharmacovigilance is a bigger domain in which PMS is one. Pharmacovigilance covers both pre and post marketing study. The PMS relies mostly on spontaneous reporting by the physicians, pharmacists and patients. Though primarily the sponsor is under obligation to carry out PMS, often the national regulatory body is too responsible for monitoring ADRs. The government of India has re-launched the National Pharmacovigilance Programme in year 2010.

It has been reported that globally more than 130 medicines have been withdrawn from various market over the last half century for various reasons due to PMS: Some examples of drugs which are withdrawn due to serious ADRs:

| Name of the drug | Indication / Pharmacology Category | Year of Marketing | Reason for withdrawal | Year of withdrawal |
|---|---|---|---|---|
| Gatifloxacin [systemic use] | Antibiotic | 1999 | Dysglycemia | 2011 |
| Rosiglitazone | Antidiabetic | 2006 | Cardiovascular Events | 2010 |
| Sibutramine | Anti-Obesity | 1998 | Cardiovascular Events | 2010 |
| Valdecoxib | Anti-inflammatory | 2001 | Cardiovascular Events | 2005 |
| Rofecoxib | Anti-Inflammatory | 1999 | Cardiovascular Events | 2004 |
| Bromfenac | Anti-inflammatory | 1997 | Serious hepatotoxic effects | 1998 (Now available for ophthalmic use) |
| Encainide | Anti- Arrhythmic Agent | 1987 | Excessive mortality | 1991 |
| Flosequinan | Vasodilator in Congestive Heart failure | 1992 | Excessive mortality | 1993 |
| Temafloxacin | Antimicrobial | 1992 | Haemolytic anaemia | 1992 |
| Benoxaprofen | Anti-inflammatory | 1982 | Liver necrosis | 1982 |
| Mibefradil | Calcium Channel Blocker for Hypertension | 1997 | Multiple drug interaction | 1998 |
| Terfenadine | Antihistamine | 1985 | Fatal cardiac arrhythmias | 1998 |
| Thalidomide | Sedative/ Hypnotic | 1957 | Phocomelia | 1961 (Now reintroduced for different indication) |

The PMS serves two primary and important goals. First, it provides a means of signal generation or the detection of new (previously unsuspected) and serious adverse drug reactions. Second, it serves to quantify the risks involved to help the drug regulating authority to take regulatory measures such as providing information or warning to prescribers or changing label of the product etc., to ensure safe and effective use of the concerned medicine.

The following principal methods are used in PMS:

***Spontaneous adverse drug reaction reporting system:*** The system requires collection and analysis of case reports of suspected adverse drug reactions. In such a system, the physicians or other healthcare professionals especially pharmacists report the ADRs in a specially designed form. The reports may be collected and analysed either at National or regional level Pharmacovigilance centres. However, the spontaneous reporting system has the limitation to provide the quantified data. The special form designed by the government of India (CDSCO) is given later in the chapter.

***Hospital based intensive monitoring:*** In the intensive monitoring systems, the trained health professionals monitor patients admitted to selected hospital wards by reviewing their clinical charts and conducting structured interviews of physicians and patients. This provides information on the extent of drug exposure and on adverse events i.e. quantification of risks. This type of system is useful for the study of acute and relatively common adverse drug reactions. The important limitations include: inability to study adequately drugs that are used mainly in out-patient care, the short follow-up period (length of stay in hospital), and the small size of the patient populations.

***Case Control studies:*** The method involves studying patients who have been affected by an adverse reaction and linking it with drug use prior to the reaction. This type of study is useful in detecting rare events or those with a long latency. It allows the calculation of an odds ratio.

***Cohort studies:*** The method requires routine data collection for signal generation and seeking correlations between extensive records of prescribing patterns for that particular drug and the occurrence of adverse events. This provides data for calculation of relative and attributable risk. Comparing with drug utilization data, it can be used as a tool for determining the extent of drug risk in the population and for developing drug regulatory decisions to keep it within reasonable bounds.

***Medical record linkage and computer data base:*** The method involves data collection from patient specific medical and pharmaceutical records. It allows a highly objective study of long term and late complications, linking well documented and validated compiled (reflow) data and equally well documented use of drugs at the individual level. It is useful for both signal generation and hypothesis testing and is inexpensive too.

The regulatory authority insists that the sponsor or the investigator should periodically furnish the periodic safety update reports (PSUR) every six months for first two years and thereafter annually for next two years. The regulatory authority may extend the period further for submitting PSUR in public interest. PSURs due for the period must be submitted within 30 days of the last day of reporting period. However, in case of serious unsuspected adverse drug reaction, reports should be submitted within 30 days of receipt of such report.

# SUSPECTED ADVERSE DRUG REACTION REPORTING FORM

For VOLUNTARY reporting of Adverse Drug Reactions by healthcare professionals

**INDIAN PHARMACOPOEIA COMMISSION**
(National Coordination Centre-Pharmacovigilance Programme of India)
Ministry of Health & Family Welfare
Government of India
Sector-23, Raj Nagar, Ghaziabad-201002
www.ipc.nic.in

**(AMC/ NCC Use only)**

AMC Report No.

Worldwide Unique

## A. PATIENT INFORMATION

1. Patient Initials ____________

2. Age at time of Event or date of birth ____________

3. Sex ☐ M ☐ F

4. Weight ____ Kgs

## B. SUSPECTED ADVERSE REACTION

5. Date of reaction started (dd/mm/yyyy)

6. Date of recovery (dd/mm/yyyy)

7. Describe reaction or problem

12. Relevant tests / laboratory data with dates

13. Other relevant history including pre-existing medical conditions (e.g. allergies, race, pregnancy, smoking, alcohol use, hepatic/ renal dysfunction etc)

14. Seriousness of the reaction

☐ Death (dd/mm/yyyy)    ☐ Congenital-anomaly
☐ Life threatening    ☐ Required intervention
☐ Hospitalization/prolonged    to prevent permanent
☐ Disability    impairment / damage
    ☐ Other (specify)

15. Outcomes

☐ Fatal    ☐ Recovering    ☐ Unknown
☐ Continuing    ☐ Recovered    ☐ Other (specify)

## C. SUSPECTED MEDICATION(S)

| S.No | 8. Name (brand and /or generic name) | Manufacturer (if known) | Batch No./ Lot No. (if known) | Exp. Date (if known)) | Dose used | Route used | Frequency | Therapy dates (if known, give duration) Date started | Date stopped | Reason for use / prescribed for |
|---|---|---|---|---|---|---|---|---|---|---|
| i. | | | | | | | | | | |
| ii. | | | | | | | | | | |
| iii. | | | | | | | | | | |
| iv. | | | | | | | | | | |

| S.No As per C | 9. Reaction abated after drug stopped or dose reduced | | | | | 10. Reaction reappeared after reintroduction | | | | |
|---|---|---|---|---|---|---|---|---|---|---|
| | Yes | No | Unknown | NA | Reduced dose | Yes | No | Unknown | NA | If reintroduced dose |
| i. | | | | | | | | | | |
| ii. | | | | | | | | | | |
| iii. | | | | | | | | | | |
| iv. | | | | | | | | | | |

11. Concomitant medical product including self medication and herbal remedies with therapy dates (exclude those used to treat reaction)

## D. REPORTER (see confidentiality section on first page)

16. Name and Professional Address : ____________________________

Pin code: __________ E-mail ____________________

Tel. No. (with STD code): ________________________

Occupation ______________ Signature ______________

17. Causality Assessment

18. Date of this report (dd/mm/yyyy)

# ADVICE ABOUT REPORTING

➢ Report adverse experiences with medications

➢ Report serious adverse reactions. A reaction is serious when the patient outcome is:
- death
- life-threatening (real risk of dying)
- hospitalization (initial or prolonged)
- disability (significant, persistent or permanent
- congenital anomaly
- required intervention to prevent permanent impairment or damage

➢ Report even if:
- You're not certain the product caused adverse reaction
- You don't have all the details, however, point nos. **1, 5, 7, 8, 11, 15, 16 & 18** (see reverse) are essentially required.

➢ Who can report:
- Any health care professional (Doctors including Dentists, Nurses and Pharmacists)

➢ Where to report:
- Please return the completed form to the nearest **Adverse drug reaction Monitoring Centre (AMC)** or to **National Coordinating Centre**
- A list of nationwide AMCs is available at: http://ipc.nic.in and also at http://cdsco.nic.in/pharmacovigilance.htm

➢ What happens to the submitted information:

- Information provided in this form is handled in strict confidence. The causality assessment is carried out at Adverse Drug Reaction Monitoring Centres (AMCs) by using WHO-UMC scale. The analyzed forms are forwarded to the National Coordinating Centre through the ADR database. Finally the data is analyzed and forwarded to the Global Pharmacovigilance Database managed by WHO Uppsala Monitoring Center in Sweden.

- The reports are periodically reviewed by the National Coordinating Centre (PvPI). The information generated on the basis of these reports helps in continuous assessment of the benefit-risk ratio of medicines.

- The information is submitted to the Steering Committee of PvPI constituted by the Ministry of Health and Family Welfare. The Committee is entrusted with the responsibility to review the data and suggest any interventions that may be required.

# Suspected Adverse Drug Reaction Reporting Form

For VOLUNTARY reporting of suspected adverse drug reactions by health care professionals

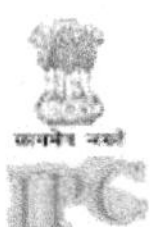

**National Coordinating Centre**
**Pharmacovigilance Programme of India**
**India Pharmacopoeia Commission**
Ministry of Health & Family Welfare
Government of India
Sector-23, Raj Nagar, Ghaziabad-201002
Tel.:0120-2783400, 2783401, 2783392,
FAX: 0120-2783313
www.ipc.nic.in

*Pharmacovigilance*
*Programme*
*of*
*India*
*for*
*Assuring Drug*
*Safety*

**Confidentiality:** The patient's identity is held in strict confidence and protected to the fullest extent. Programme staff is not ex-pected to and will not disclose the reporter's identity in response to a request from the public. Submission of a report does not constitute an admission that medical personnel or manufacturer or the product caused or contributed to the reaction.

## Key Points to Remember

- The clinical trials are human experimentations done in an attempt to evaluate the safety and efficacy of an investigational product.

- There are three important characteristics of a clinical trial design: controls, randomization and blinding.

- There are three common types of designs: parallel group design, cross over design, and factorial design. Randomized controlled trials are accepted currently as gold standard.

- Schedule Y of Drugs and Cosmetics Rules is the guiding force for clinical trial: submission of application to approval and conducting the trial. DCGI is the licensing authority for issuing permission to conduct clinical trials.

- Responsibilities of stake holders:
  - Regulatory Authority: Approval of trials, ensuring the trial is conducted as per GCP and Indian guidelines, and ensuring payment of compensation in case of trial related injury.
  - Sponsor: Responsible for quality assurance system, complying with GCP requirements and payment of compensation in trial related injury.
  - Investigator: Conducting the trial as per approved protocol and GCP guidelines.
  - Ethics Committee: Responsible to safe guard the rights, safety and well beings of the study participants. EC is empowered to approve the study protocol, approve the study site and approving number of trials to which one investigator can take up at a time.

- Informed Consent Form: Informed consent is to be obtained before enrolling the participants. The form is to be prepared as per the requirements of schedule Y. This must contain information related to compensation in trial related injury.

- The clinical trial has four phases:
  - Phase – I: Human Pharmacology – usually in healthy human volunteers to determine the pharmacokinetic data

and maximum tolerated dose. For anticancer drugs, this is done in cancer patients.

  o Phase – II: Therapeutic Exploratory Trials – in patients to evaluate the effectiveness, and to determine the dose and dosage regimen for phase – III study.

  o Phase – III: Therapeutic Confirmatory Trials – is designed in patients to confirm the preliminary evidence accumulated in phase II that the drug is safe and effective, intended indication and recipient population. The data generated becomes the basis for getting marketing approval.

  o Phase – IV: Post Marketing Trials – the study is continued after marketing approval for optimizing the drug use and collecting more safety information and information support for off label use.

- The Post Marketing Surveillance is the safety monitoring of approved drugs while they are in market. The marketing company needs to submit periodic safety update reports every six months for first two years and then on yearly basis for next two years.

- The registration of clinical trial is mandatory. The investigator or the primary sponsor can register based on the mutual agreement. The primary sponsor is accountable.

- The Drugs and Cosmetics Act, and the rules specify the conditions of import and manufacture of drugs for examination, test or analysis.

- The methodologies for PMS Study: spontaneous adverse drug reaction reporting system, hospital based intensive monitoring, case control studies, cohort studies, medical record linkage and computer data base.

- In trial related injury including death, the study participant or nominee is entitled for financial compensation over above the medical care.  The maximum compensation is now fixed at Rs. 8 lakh.

# CHAPTER 5

# Ethical Issues in Clinical Research

"Ethics is knowing the difference between what you have the right to do and what is right to do"

-Potter Stewart

---

**After reading this chapter, you should be able to know or learn:**

- Basic principles of ethics;
- Milestones in development of ethical guidelines;
- Salient points of ICMR's guidelines;
- Constitution of Institutional Ethics Committee;
- SOP for functioning of IEC;
- Some infamous unethical human experimentations; and
- Understand how to develop inform consent form.

---

An experiment is done to discover or to test a supposition or principle and it does not ensure the outcome. The experiment always has a chance and because of this chance the experimentation on human beings invites a serious attention of ethics. The basic principle is to safeguard the interest of the human subjects participating in clinical research. The four basic underlying principles are:

1. *Beneficence:* This requires that good should result, harm should be avoided, or that benefits should justify the risk or harm;

2. *Non-Maleficence*: Do no harm;

3. *Respect for rights (autonomy):* This requires that the research subject should have free choice whether to participate or not and protection for those with diminished autonomy; and

4. *Justice:* This requires an equal distribution of burden and benefit.

As on January 2005, it is mandatory for clinical trials to comply with Indian Council for Medical Research's (ICMR) ethical guidelines for biomedical research on humans  and the World Medical Association' Declaration of Helsinki. The declaration of Helsinki is accepted as an international standard for biomedical research.

***Development of Ethical Guidelines in India:***

1. The ethical codes of conduct for medical professionals and physicians existed since ancient times. *Charaka Samhita* of Ayurveda describes the duties of physicians towards their patients and other fellow professionals. Similar code is also described in *Susruta Samhita* for surgeons.

2. In 1980 the ICMR issued a "Policy Statement on Ethical Considerations for Research on Human Subjects".

3. ICMR set up the Justice Venkatachaliah Committee in 1996 to update 1980 guideline.

4. The ICMR released the revised guideline "Ethical Guidelines for Biomedical Research on Human Subject" in 2000.

5. The ICMR Guideline was revised in 2006.

6. Guidelines for Stem Cell Research and Therapy in 2007.

7. Registration of Ethics Committee is mandatory: made in 2013.

8. Draft National Ethical Guidelines for Biomedical and Health Research involving Human Participants: released by ICMR in 2016.

***Development of International Ethical Guidelines:***

1. The ethical codes of conduct for medical professionals and physicians existed since ancient times. 'Hippocratic Oath' of the Greco – Roman Period emphasizing on 'Do No Harm'.

2. Post Second World War (1939-45): The trial of German Medical Practitioners (in Nuremberg Military Tribunal's Meeting) were accused of conducting experiments on human participants

without their consent and exposing them to grave risk of death or permanent impairment of their faculties. This raised worldwide concern. Some of the brutalities performed includes high altitude experiments, freezing experiments, poison experiments, phosphorous burns and chemical sterilization.

3. Development of Nuremberg Code (1947) – Ten basic principles for medical research that must be observed to satisfy moral, ethical and legal concepts. This highlighted the essentiality of voluntary consent.

4. Universal Declaration of Human Rights adopted in UN General Assembly in 1948 expressing concern about the rights of human beings subjected to involuntary maltreatment.

5. Helsinki Declaration (1964) – In association with Council for International Organizations of Medical Sciences (CIOMS), the World Medical Association (WMA) formulated general principles on use of human subjects in medical research in addition to specific guidelines for biomedical research. This has been periodically revised.

6. International Covenant on Civil and Political Rights (1966) – This specifically stated that no one shall be subjected to torture or to cruelty or degrading treatment or punishment. In particular, no one shall be subjected without his consent to medical or scientific treatment.

7. Belmont Report (1979) – The Tuskegee Syphilis Study had a wide repercussion that forced the US government to establish the National Commission for the Protection of Human Subjects of Biomedical and Behavioural Research  leading to Belmont Report. This is the first National Guidelines for Medical Research in USA.

8. WHO and CIOMS (1982) drafted the proposed International Guidelines for Biomedical Research involving Human Subjects.

9. CIOMS (1991) released the International Guidelines for Ethical Review in Epidemiological Studies.

10. CIOMS (1993) – International Ethical Guidelines for Biomedical research involving Human Subjects was released.

11. The Universal Declaration on Human Genome and Human Rights (1997).

12. The International Declaration on Human Gene Data (2003).

13. The Universal Declaration on Bioethics and Human Rights (2005).

14. The revision of Helsinki Declaration (2008) – This strongly discourages the use of placebo controlled trials when a treatment exists.

15. Helsinki declaration was revised [50th Anniversary revision] in 2014:

    • Provision of compensation and treatment of research related injuries – the research participants should not bear the cost of treatment.

    • Emphasis on dissemination of research results including studies with negative results – should increase the value of medical research.

Though the declaration of Helsinki remains the backbone of National Ethical guidelines, even after the several revisions, it is not above criticism: it mainly addresses physicians (not other health workforce), no provision for possibility of waiving consent for some research etc..

An increasing number of reports have been appearing in press highlighting the unethical and illegal practices that exploit people's social and economic vulnerability, subject them to serious risk without their knowledge and consent, and do not even assure them of access to the drugs developed from the trials. The government is planning to mandate biometric identification for clinical trial volunteers in the country to bring in global standards and weed out unethical practices. Unlike other forms of identification, biometric identification which relies on the unique physical characteristics of a person, like the iris of the eye or a fingerprint is almost impossible to fudge.

The ICMR statement of Ethical Guidelines for Biomedical Research on Human Subjects is known as ICMR Code. The statement is divided into: General Principles on Research and Specific Principles on Research - in specific areas of biomedical research. Though it covers the following specific principles of research: Clinical Evaluation of Drugs / Devices / Diagnostics / Vaccines / Herbal Remedies, Epidemiological Studies, Human Genetics and Genomics Research, Research in Transplantation, and Assisted Reproductive Technologies, the present text restricts its discussion to clinical evaluation of drugs in addition to the general principles of ethics. The salient points are only mentioned and the readers are encouraged to look at the original guideline for more details.

*Research on human beings must necessarily ensure that*

  (i) The **PURPOSE** of research is directed towards the increase of knowledge about the human condition in relation to its social and natural environment and the research is for the betterment of all, especially the least advantaged.

  (ii) The research is **CONDUCTED** under conditions that the participants are treated in a manner conducive to and consistent with their dignity and well being  and after ensuring the well being of the participant in question.

  (iii) The research must be subjected to a regime of **EVALUATION** at all stages of the proposal ranging from research design and experimentation to the use of the results ensuring the safety of each human life.

## Statement of General Principles

*Research on human beings needs to follow the 12 principles given below:*

  (i) **Principles of essentiality:** The research must be absolutely essential as considered by an appropriate and responsible body of persons who are external to the particular research. The research is necessary for the advancement of knowledge and for the benefit of all members of the human species and for the ecological and environmental well being of the planet.

  (ii) **Principles of voluntariness, informed consent and community agreement:** The research participants must be apprised of the impact and risk involved and their right to participate or abstain from participation at any time. It is necessary to obtain the informed consent from the participants. Where the informed consent is not possible from the participant, it must be obtained from someone who is empowered to act on their behalf. They need to be continually kept informed of any and all developments as they affect them and others.

  (iii) **Principles of non-exploitation:** The research participants are to be remunerated for their involvement in research and are to be made fully apprised of all the dangers arising in and out of the research. The research should have an in-built mechanism for compensation for the human participants either through insurance cover or any other appropriate means to cover all foreseeable and unforeseeable risks.

**(iv) Principles of privacy and confidentiality:** The    identity and records of participants of the research are as far as possible kept confidential; and that no details about identity of human participants would be disclosed without valid scientific and legal reasons.

**(v) Principles of precaution and risk minimization:** Due care and caution should be taken at all stages of the research and experiment (from its inception to its applicative use) to ensure that the research participant and those affected by it including community are put to the minimum risk, suffer from no known irreversible adverse effects.

**(vi) Principles of professional competence:** The research is to be conducted at all times by competent and qualified persons who act with total integrity and impartiality and who have been made aware of the ethical considerations to be borne in mind in respect of research.

**(vii) Principles of accountability and transparency:** The research is to be conducted in a fair, honest, impartial and transparent manner. All associated with the research must make full disclosure with respect to their interest in the research, and any conflict of interest that may exist. Full and complete records of the research inclusive of data and notes are to be retained for reasonable period as may be required for various purposes including for scrutiny by the appropriate legal and administrative authority, if necessary.

**(viii) Principles of the maximisation of the public interest and of distributive justice:** The outcome of the research must have use to benefit for all kind of people and not just those who are socially better off.

**(ix) Principles of institutional arrangements:** The people connected with research must ensure that all procedures adopted are in transparent manner and ensure that research reports, materials and data connected with the research are duly preserved and archived.

**(x) Principles of public domain:** The research and emanating from such research must be brought into the public domain so that its results are generally made known through scientific and other publications subject to such rights as are available.

**(xi) Principles of totality of responsibility:** All persons or groups associated with the research in various capacities must have the professional and moral responsibility, for the due observance of all the principles, guidelines or prescriptions laid down generally. The effect of the research or experiment is duly monitored and constantly subject to review and remedial action at all stages of the research and experiment and its future use.

**(xii) Principles of compliance:** The persons conducting or associated with the research must ensure that both the letter and the spirit of these guidelines, as well as any other norms, directions and guidelines are scrupulously observed and duly complied.

---

**Landmark Ethical Clearance [Hindu, August 25, 2014]:**

The World Health Organization panel unanimously agreed on 14th August 2014 for use of "unproven interventions" in humans as potential treatment or prevention options for the Ebola virus disease. This is accepted to be ethical to use this intervention in the West African countries of Liberia, Guinea, Sierra Leone and Nigeria. The controversy aroused over the use of an untested drug, ZMapp, on two Americans who came down with the disease that forced the WHO to look into the ethics of using it in the these four countries.

Prior to the WHO clearance, three main reasons were cited for not supplying the untested drug to dying Africans: non-availability of mechanism to monitor serious adverse effects; the inability of the U.S. to decide who the recipients of a limited supply of drugs should be; and the backlash the drug company and the U.S. would face if the experimental drug first used on Africans were to cause serious adverse effects.

---

## Ethical Review Procedures

The research proposal must be cleared by an appropriately constituted Institutional Ethics Committee (IEC), also referred to as Institutional Review Board (IRB), Ethics Review Board (ERB) and Research Ethics Board (REB) in other countries, to safeguard the welfare and the rights of the participants. The independent ethics committees [IEC (Ind)] functioning outside institutions can approve proposals of those researchers who have no institutional attachments or work in institutions with no ethics committee.

**Basic Responsibilities of Ethics Committee:** The IEC needs to ensure the appropriateness of the proposal through appropriate scientific review committee and also to ensure the competent review of the ethical aspects. Ethics Committee has a continuing responsibility of regular monitoring of the approved programmes to foresee the compliance of the ethics during the period of the project. Such an ongoing review shall be in accordance with the international guidelines and the Standard Operating Procedures (SOP) of the WHO available at www.who.int. The IECs should specify in writing the authority under which the Committee is established.

Small institutions could form alliance with other IECs or approach registered IEC (Ind). Large institutions/Universities with large number of proposals can have more than one suitably constituted IECs for different research areas for which large number of research proposals are submitted. However, the institutional policy should be same for all these IECs to safeguard the research participant's rights.

A sub-committee of the main IEC may review proposals submitted by undergraduate or post-graduate students. The responsibilities of an IEC can be defined as follows:

1. To protect the dignity, rights and well being of the potential research participants.
2. To ensure that universal ethical values and international scientific standards are expressed in terms of local community values and customs.
3. To assist in the development and the education of a research community responsive to local health care requirements.

There have been a sea change on the **responsibilities and functioning** of Ethics Committees [with amendment of Drugs and Cosmetics Rules 2013]:

- The ECs need to register with DCGI. No EC can review and accord its approval to a clinical trial protocol without prior registration with DCGI;
- The prime responsibility is to safe guard the rights, safety and well-being of research participants;
- All ECs should function in compliance with the regulations and GCP guidance for composition, quorum, training, review process, safety review, continue monitoring over sight and documentation;
- EC decides the number of trials an investigator can have at a time (previously it was restricted only 3 trials per investigator);
- EC decides the place of trials – which hospital can be approved (previously there was restriction-only hospitals with minimum of 50 beds were permissible);
- EC can decide adding new investigator or new site for clinical trial. There is no need of no objection certificate from DCGI. However,

applicant has to inform the DCGI about such additions or deletions. If no objection is received thereafter, it would be of deemed to have concurrence of CDSCO.

- The EC members need to be conversant with the provisions of clinical trials under schedule Y, Indian GCP guidelines, and other regulatory requirements to carry out their responsibilities;

- Following the approval, the EC has to oversee and monitor the clinical trials being conducted at regular intervals and take appropriate actions in case of non-compliance to the conditions of trial approval; and

- The EC needs to analyse and forward its opinion to CDSCO in the case of any serious adverse event (SAE) occurring to the trial subjects as per the compensation rule. The investigator and sponsor are required to submit a follow up report of SAE within 14 calendar days to the EC and CDSCO. The EC needs to submit its opinion on the relationship between the SAE and clinical trial. The readers may refer to Clinical Trials chapter for more details on compensation.

- EC is open for inspection by CDSCO (or with State Drugs Control) Officers. The officers may verify the compliance to the requirements of schedule Y, GCP guidelines and other relevant regulations for safeguarding the rights, safety and well-being of the trial subjects.

## Registration of EC

Every EC needs to be registered with DCGI in order to review and accord approval of clinical trials. EC needs to apply to the Licensing Authority (DCGI) in accordance with the requirements as specified in Appendix VIII of schedule Y. Please refer Appendix B for more details.

The registration is valid for a period of three years unless suspended or cancelled. If the application for re-registration is received before three months of expiry of registration, the registration will continue in force till further orders. The licensing authority has the power to cancel or suspend the registration for the period as appropriate after giving a 'show cause' notice. EC, whose registration is cancelled or suspended, will have opportunity to appeal before the Government within ninety days of receipt of suspension or cancellation order. The central government, after giving an opportunity to defend, may confirm, reverse or modify such order.

**Information required to be submitted by the Applicant for Registration**

1. Name of the ethics committee;
2. Authority under which EC is constituted, membership requirement. Terms of reference, conditions of appointment and the quorum required;
3. The procedure for resignation, replacement or removal of the members;
4. Address of the ethics committee;
5. Name, address, qualification, organizational title, telephone number, fax, e-mail, mailing address and brief profile of the chairman;
6. Names, qualifications, organizational titles, telephone number, fax number, e-mail, and mailing address of the members. The information should also include member's specialty: primary, scientific or non-scientific, member's affiliation with the institution, and patient group representation, if any;
7. Details of the supporting staff;
8. The standard operating procedure to be followed by the EC in general;
9. The standard operating procedures to be followed by the EC for vulnerable populations;
10. Policy regarding training for new and existing members along with standard operating procedures;
11. Policy to monitor and avoid conflict of interest with SOP; and
12. If the committee has been audited or inspected previously, furnish the details.

## Composition of IEC

The Ethics committee is a committee consisting of medical, scientific, non-medical, non-scientific members. Its primary responsibility is to ensure protection of rights, safety and well-being of the clinical trial subjects.

The IECs should be multidisciplinary and multi-sectorial in composition. Independence and competence are the two hallmarks of an IEC. The number of persons in an ethics committee should be kept fairly small. It is generally accepted that a minimum of five persons is required to form the quorum without which a decision regarding the research should not be taken.

1. EC should have at least seven members. One member who is from outside the institute is the chairperson. One member is the member secretary. Other members should be from scientific, medical, non-medical and non-scientific fields including lay public.

2. It should have at least one member whose primary area of interest or specialisation is non-scientific and at least one member who is independent of the institution. There should be appropriate gender representation.

3. The EC can have its members from other institutions or communities, if necessary.

4. For review of each protocol, the quorum of ethics committee should have at least five members consisting of:
   (a) Basic medical scientist (preferably pharmacologist);
   (b) Clinician;
   (c) Legal expert;
   (d) Social scientist or representative of non-government voluntary agency or philosopher or ethicist or theologian or similar person; and
   (e) Lay person from the community.

5. The members representing medical scientists or clinicians must have post graduate qualification and adequate experience in the respective fields. They should be aware of their roles and responsibilities.

6. As far as possible specific patient group should be represented in the Committee based on the research areas such as HIV, genetic disorder etc.

7. There should not be conflict of interest. The members should withdraw voluntarily while making a decision giving in writing about the conflict of interest. Every member has to sign a declaration on conflict of interest.

8. Subject experts or other experts may be invited to the meeting seeking their advice. They would have no voting rights.

## Terms of Reference for Operation of IEC

Every IEC should have its own written SOPs according to which the Committee should function. The SOP should specify the terms of appointment with reference to the duration of the term, the policy for removal, replacement, resignation procedure, frequency of meetings, and payment of processing fee to the IEC for review, honorarium/ consultancy to the members/ invited experts *etc.*

The SOPs should be updated periodically based on the changing requirements. The term of appointment of members could be extended for another term and a defined percentage of members could be changed on regular basis. It would be preferable to appoint persons trained in bioethics or persons conversant with ethical guidelines and laws of the country. Substitute member may be nominated if meetings have been continuously missed by a member due to illness or other unforeseen circumstances. For this the criteria for number of missed meetings may be defined in the SOP.

**Independent Ethics Committees** are empowered to review and approve only the study protocols and related documents of BA/BE studies of approved drug molecules and also carry ongoing review of such studies. They are not empowered to review and approve new clinical trials.

**Standard Operating Procedures (SOPs) for Institutional Ethics Committee (IEC) of ICMR's Headquarters Office, New Delhi: [http://icmr.nic.in/bioethics/bioethics%20cell/SOP_of_IEC.pdf].**

*This is an example of SOP for EC.*

1. **Objective:** The objective of this SOP is to contribute to the effective functioning of the IEC at the Indian Council of Medical Research, Headquarters Office, New Delhi, India, so that a quality and consistent ethical review mechanism for health and biomedical research is put in place for all proposals dealt by the Committee.

2. **Role of IEC ICMR Headquarters IEC will review research proposals involving human subjects submitted by scientists of ICMR Headquarters Office, New Delhi, to various funding or other agencies for grant of funds or technical collaboration at the ICMR Headquarters office at New Delhi.**

   All the 26 Institutes under ICMR have their own institutional ethics committees to review the projects undertaken by them for research. ICMR Headquarters IEC will review and approve all types of research proposals involving human participants with a view to safeguard the dignity, rights, safety and well-being of all actual or potential research participants. The goals of research, however important, should never be permitted to override the health and well-being of the research subjects.

The IEC will take care that all the cardinal principles of research ethics viz. Autonomy, Beneficence, Non- maleficience and Justice. For this purpose, it will look into the aspects of informed consent process, risk benefit ratio, distribution of burden and benefit and provisions for appropriate compensations wherever required. It will review the proposals before start of the studies as well as monitor the research throughout the study until and after completion by examining the annual reports and final reports. The committee will also examine whether all regulatory requirements and laws are complied with or not.

3.  **Composition of IEC:**
    1.  Chairman
    2.  A Basic Scientist
    3.  Two Clinicians
    4.  A Lawyer
    5.  A Social Scientist
    6.  A Philosopher
    7.  A lay Person
    8.  Member Secretary.

4.  **Authority under which IEC is constituted:** The Director-General of ICMR, New Delhi, constitutes ICMR's Headquarters, IEC.

5.  **Membership requirements:**
    (a)  The members are appointed by the DG, ICMR.
    (b)  The members are drawn from different Institutes, and specialties to give a multisectorial, multidimensional structure.
    (c)  The duration of appointment is initially for a period of 3 years
    (d)  At the end of 3 years, the committee is reconstituted, and 50% of the members will be replaced.
    (e)  A member can be replaced in the event of death or long-term assignments outside the country or for any misconduct deemed unfit for a member.
    (f)  A member can tender resignation from the committee with proper reasons to do so, which should be acceptable to the DG, ICMR.
    (g)  All members should maintain absolute confidentiality of all discussions during the meeting.

6. **Quorum requirements:** The minimum of 50% + 1 member are required to compose a quorum.

   All decisions should be taken in meetings and not by circulation of project proposals.

7. **Offices:** The Chairperson will conduct all meetings of the IEC. If for reasons beyond control, the Chairperson is not available, an alternate Chairperson will be nominated by the DG from the members present, who will conduct the meeting.

   The Member Secretary is responsible for organizing the meetings, maintaining the records and communicating with all concerned. He/she will prepare the minutes of the meetings and get it approved by the Chairman before communicating to the researchers with the approval of the DG, ICMR.

8. **Independent consultants:** IEC may call upon subject experts as independent consultants who may provide special review of selected research protocols, if needed. These experts may be specialists in ethical or legal aspects, specific diseases or methodologies, or represent specific communities, patient groups or special interest groups e.g. Cancer patients, HIV/AIDS positive persons or ethnic minorities. They are required to give their specialized views but do not take part in the decision making process which will be made by the members of the IEC.

9. **Applications Procedures:**
   (a) All proposals are to be submitted in the prescribed application form, the details of which are given under Documentation
   (b) All relevant documents to be enclosed with application form
   (c) 12 copies of the proposal along with the application in prescribed format to be submitted duly forwarded by the Head of the Division.
   (d) The date of meeting will be intimated to the researcher, to be present, if necessary to offer clarifications.
   (e) The decision will be communicated in writing. If revision is to be made, the revised document in 12 copies need to be submitted before the next meeting.

10. **Documentation:** For a thorough and complete review, all research proposals are to be submitted with the following documents:
    1. Name of the applicant with designation
    2. Name of the Institute/ Hospital / Field area where research will be conducted.

3.  Approval of the Head of the Division
4.  Protocol of the proposed research
5.  Ethical issues in the study and plans to address these issues.
6.  Proformae, questionnaires, follow up card, etc.
7.  Patient information sheet and informed consent form in local language.
8.  For any drug / device trial, all relevant pre-clinical animal data and clinical trial data from other countries, if available.
9.  Statement describing compensation for study subjects for participation and/or study related injuries.
10. Curriculum vitae of all the investigators with relevant publications in last five years.
11. Any regulatory clearances required.
12. Source of funding and financial requirements for the project.
13. An agreement to report any serious side effects or adverse drug reactions to IEC.
14. Statement of conflicts of interest, if any.
15. Any other information relevant to the study.

**11. Review procedures:**

(a) The meeting of the IEC will be held as and when the proposals are received for review. However, if need be, meetings can be held at scheduled intervals when large number of proposals are to be reviewed..

(b) The proposals will be sent to members at least 3 weeks in advance.

(c) Decisions will be taken by consensus after discussions.

(d) Researchers will be invited to offer clarifications if need be.

(e) Independent consultants/Experts will be invited to offer their opinion on specific research proposals.

(f) The decisions will be minuted and Chairperson's approval will be taken in writing.

**12. Element of review:**

(a) Scientific design and conduct of the study.
(b) Approval of appropriate scientific review committees.
(c) Examination of predictable risks/harms.

   (d)  Examination of potential benefits.

   (e)  Procedure for selection of subjects: Exclusion / Inclusion criteria

   (f)  Management of research related injuries, side effects, ADRs.

   (g)  Compensation provisions.

   (h)  Justification for placebo in control arm, if any.

   (i)  Availability of products after the study, if applicable.

   (j)  Patient information sheet and informed consent form in local language.

   (k)  Protection of privacy and confidentiality.

   (l)  Involvement of the community, wherever necessary.

   (m)  Plans for data analysis and reporting

   (n)  Adherence to all regulatory requirements

13. **Expedited/Interim review:** All revised proposals, unless specifically required to go to the main committee, will be examined in a meeting of identified members convened by the Chairman to expedite decision making. Such expedited review may also be taken up in cases of nationally relevant proposals requiring urgent review

14. **Decision-making:**

   (a)  Members will discuss the various issues before arriving at a consensus decision.

   (b)  Decisions will be made only in meetings where quorum is complete.

   (c)  Only members can make the decision. The expert consultants will only offer their opinions.

   (d)  Decision may be to approve, reject or modify the proposals. Specific suggestions should be given for modifications.

   (e)  Modified proposals may be reviewed by an interim review through identified members.

   (f)  Negative decisions should always be substantiated by appropriate reasons.

15. **Communicating the decision:**

    (a) Decision will be communicated by the Member Secretary in writing.

    (b) Suggestions of IEC, if any, should be sent for modifications.

    (c) Reasons for rejection should be informed to the researchers. There is no need to communicate the name of the specific expert or member who made the review.

16. **Follow up procedures:**

    (a) Regular reports should be submitted for regular review.

    (b) Final report to be submitted at the end of study.

    (c) Any serious side effects, adverse drug reactions and the interventions undertaken to be intimated.

    (d) Protocol deviation, if any, to be informed with adequate justifications.

    (e) Any new information related to the study should be communicated.

    (f) Premature termination of study should be notified with reasons and summary of the studies done so far.

17. **Archiving/Record keeping:**

    (a) Curriculum Vitae (CV) of all members of IEC.

    (b) Copy of all study protocols with enclosed documents, annual reports, side-effects/ADRS etc.

    (c) Minutes of all meetings with due signature of Chairperson.

    (d) Copy of all existing national and international guidelines on research ethics.

    (e) Copy of all correspondence with members, researchers and other regulatory bodies.

    (f) Final report of the approved projects.

18. **Updating IEC members:**

    (a) All relevant new guidelines to be brought to the attention of the members.

    (b) Members should be encouraged to attend national and international training programs in research ethics for maintaining quality in ethical review and to be aware of the latest developments in this area.

## Maintenance of Records

All documentation and communication of an ethics committee must be dated, filed and preserved. Strict confidentiality must be maintained while accessing and retrieving the documents. Following records are required to be maintained:

- The constitution and composition of the EC;
- The CV of all committee members;
- SOPs followed by the committee;
- National and International guidelines;
- Copies of the protocol, data collection formats, case report forms, investigator's brochures, etc. submitted for review;
- All correspondences with committee members and investigator regarding application, decision and follow up;
- Agenda of all ethics committee meetings;
- Minutes of all ethics committee meeting with signature of chairman;
- Copies of decisions communicated to the applicants;
- Record of all notifications issued for premature termination of a study with a summary of reasons;
- Final report of the study including microfilms, compact disks, or video recordings.

All records, hard and soft copies, should be safely maintained for a period of at least five years after termination or completion of the trials.

## Review Procedure of Research Proposal

The IEC should review every research proposal before the research is initiated. It should ensure that a scientific evaluation has been completed before ethical review is taken up. The Committee should evaluate the possible risks to the participants with proper justification, the expected benefits and adequacy of documentation for ensuring privacy, confidentiality and the justice issues.

The IEC's member-secretary or secretariat shall screen the proposals for their completeness and depending on the risk involved categorise them into three types, namely, **exemption from review, expedited review** and **full review**. These terms are explained below.

*Minimal risk:* The risk may be anticipated as harm or discomfort not greater than that encountered in routine daily life activities of general popula tion or during the performance of routine physical or psychological examinations or tests. However, in some cases like surgery, chemotherapy or radiation therapy, great risk would be inherent in the treatment itself, but this may be within the range of minimal risk for the research participant undergoing these interventions since it would be undertaken as part of current every day life. All proposals will be scrutinised to decide under which of the following three categories it will be considered:

1. **Exemption from Review:** Proposals which present less than minimal risk fall under this category as seen in following situation: Research on educational practices such as instructional strategies or effectiveness of or the comparison among instructional techniques, curricula, or classroom management methods.

   **Exceptions**

   - When research on use of educational tests, survey or interview procedures, or observation of public behavior can identify the human participant directly or through identifiers, and the disclosure of information outside research could subject the participant to the risk of civil or criminal or financial liability or psychosocial harm.

   - When interviews involve direct approach or access to private papers.

2. **Expedited Review:** The proposals presenting no more than minimal risk to research participants may be subjected to expedited review. The Member- Secretary and the Chairperson of the IEC or designated member of the Committee or Subcommittee of the IEC may do expedited review only if the protocols involve

   1. Minor deviations from originally approved research during the period of approval (usually of one year duration).

   2. Revised proposal previously approved through full review by the IEC or continuing review of approved proposals where there is no additional risk or activity is limited to data analysis.

   3. Research activities that involve only procedures listed in one or more of the following categories:

*Clinical studies of drugs and medical devices only when:*

   (i)  Research is on already approved drugs except when studying drug interaction or conducting trial on vulnerable population or

  (ii)  Adverse Event (AE) or unexpected Adverse Drug Reaction (ADR) of minor nature is reported.

4. Research involving clinical materials (data, documents, records, or specimens) that have been collected for non-research (clinical) purposes.

5. When in emergency situations like serious outbreaks or disasters a full review of the research is not possible, prior written permission of IEC may be taken before use of the test intervention. Such research can only be approved for pilot study or preliminary work to study the safety and efficacy of the intervention and **the same participants should not be included** in the clinical trial that may be initiated later based on the findings of the pilot study.

  **(a)**  **Research on interventions in emergency situation:** When proven prophylactic, diagnostic, and therapeutic methods do not exist or have been ineffective, physicians may use new intervention as investigational drug (IND) / devices/ vaccine to provide emergency medical care to their patients in life threatening conditions. Research in such instance of medical care could be allowed in patients –

     (i)  When consent of person/ patient/ responsible relative or custodian/ team of designated doctors for such an event are not possible. However, information about the intervention should be given to the relative/ legal guardian when available later;

    (ii)  When the intervention has undergone testing for safety prior to its use in emergency situations and sponsor has obtained prior approval of DCGI;

   (iii)  Only if the local IEC reviews the protocol since institutional responsibility is of paramount importance in such instances;

   (iv)  If Data Safety Monitoring Board (DSMB) is constituted to review the data.

  **(b)**  **Research on disaster management:** It may be unethical sometimes not to do research in disasters. Disasters create vulnerable persons and groups in society, particularly so in disadvantaged communities, and therefore, the following points need to be considered when reviewing such research:

(i) Research planned to be conducted after a disaster should be essential culturally sensitive and specific in nature with possible application in future disaster situations.

(ii) Disaster-affected community participation before and during the research is essential and its representative or advocate must be identified.

(iii) Extra care must be taken to protect the privacy and confidentiality of participants and communities.

(iv) Protection must be ensured so that only minimal additional risk is imposed.

(v) The research undertaken should provide direct or indirect benefits to the participants, the disaster-affected community or future disaster- affected population and *a priori* agreement should be reached on this, whenever possible, between the community and the researcher.

(vi) All international collaborative research in the disaster-affected area should be done with a local partner on an equal partnership basis.

(vii) Transfer of biological material, if any, should be as per Government rules taking care of intellectual property rights issues.

3. **Full Review:** All research presenting with more than minimal risk, proposals/ protocols which do not qualify for exempted or expedited review and projects that involve vulnerable population and special groups shall be subjected to full review by all the members. While reviewing the proposals, the following situations may be carefully assessed against the existing facilities at the research site for risk/benefit analysis:

(a) **Collection of blood samples** by finger prick, heel prick, ear prick, or venipuncture:

(i) From healthy adults and non-pregnant women who weigh normal for their age and not more than 500 ml blood is drawn in an 8 week period and frequency of collection is not more than 2 times per week;

(ii) From other adults and children, where the age, weight, and health of the participants, the collection procedure, the amount of blood to be collected, and the frequency with which it will be collected has been considered and not more than 50 ml or 3 ml per kg, whichever is lesser is drawn in an 8 week period and not more than 2 times per week;

(iii) From neonates depending on the haemodynamics and, body weight of the baby- not more than 10% of blood is drawn within 48 – 72 hours. If more than this amount is to be drawn it becomes a risky condition requiring infusion/blood transfusion;

(iv) Prospective collection of biological specimens for research purposes by noninvasive means. For instance:

1. Skin appendages like hair and nail clippings in a non-disfiguring manner;

2. Dental procedures-deciduous teeth at time of exfoliation or if routine patient care indicates a need for extraction of permanent teeth; supra and sub-gingival dental plaque and calculus, provided the collection procedure is not more invasive than routine prophylactic scaling of the teeth;

3. Excreta and external secretions (including sweat);

4. Uncannulated saliva collected either in an unstimulated fashion or stimulated by chewing gum or by applying a dilute citric solution to the tongue;

5. Placenta removed at delivery;

6. Amniotic fluid obtained at the time of rupture of the membrane prior to or during labor;

7. Mucosal and skin cells collected by buccal scraping or swab, skin swab, or mouth washings;

8. Sputum collected after saline mist nebulization and bronchial lavages.

**(b) Collection of data through noninvasive procedures** routinely employed in clinical practice. Where medical devices are employed, they must be cleared/ approved for marketing, for instance-

(i) Physical sensors that are applied either to the surface of the body or at a distance and do not involve input of significant amounts of energy into the participant or an invasion of the participant's privacy;

(ii) Weighing or testing sensory acuity;

(iii) Magnetic resonance imaging;

(iv) electrocardiography, echocardiography, electroencephalography, thermography, detection of naturally occurring radioactivity, electroretinography, ultrasound, diagnostic infrared imaging, doppler blood flow;

(v) Moderate exercise, muscular strength testing, body composition assessment, and flexibility testing where appropriate given the age, weight, and health of the individual.

**(c) Research involving clinical materials** (data, documents, records, or specimens) that will be collected solely for non-research (clinical) purposes.

**(d) Collection of data** from voice, video, digital, or image recordings made for research purposes.

**(e) Research** on individual or group characteristics or behaviours not limited to research on perception, cognition, motivation, identity, language, communication, cultural beliefs or practices, and social behaviour or research employing survey, interview, oral history, focus group, program evaluation, human factors evaluation, or quality assurance methodologies.

## Decision Making Process

The IEC should be able to provide complete and adequate review of the research proposals submitted to them. It should meet periodically at frequent intervals to review new proposals, evaluate annual progress of ongoing ones, review serious adverse event (SAE) reports and assess final reports of all research activities involving human beings through a previously scheduled agenda, amended wherever appropriate. The following points should be considered while doing so:

1. The decision must be taken by a broad consensus after the quorum requirements are fulfilled to recommend / reject / suggest modification for a repeat review or advice appropriate steps. The Member Secretary should communicate the decision in writing to the Principal Investigator.

2. If a member has conflict-of-interest (COI) involving a project then s/he should submit this in writing to the chairperson before the review meeting, and it should also be recorded in the minutes.

3. If one of the members has her/his own proposal for review or has any COI then s/he should withdraw from the IEC while the project is being discussed.

4. A negative decision should always be supported by clearly defined reasons.

5. An IEC may decide to reverse its positive decision on a study if it receives information that may adversely affect the risk/ benefit ratio.

6. The discontinuation of a trial should be ordered if the IEC finds that the goals of the trial have already been achieved midway or unequivocal results are obtained.

7. In case of premature termination of study, notification should include the reasons for termination along with the summary of results conducted till date.

8. The following circumstances require the matter to be brought to the attention of IEC:

    (a) any amendment to the protocol from the originally approved protocol with proper justification;

    (b) serious and unexpected adverse events and remedial steps taken to tackle them;

    (c) any new information that may influence the conduct of the study.

9. If necessary, the applicant/investigator may be invited to present the protocol or offer clarifications in the meeting. Representative of the patient groups or interest groups can be invited during deliberations to offer their viewpoint.

10. Subject experts may be invited to offer their views, but should not take part in the decision making process. However, her / his opinion must be recorded.

11. Minutes of the meetings are to be approved and signed by the Chairperson/ alternate Chairperson/ designated member of the committee.

## Review Process

The method of review should be stated in the SOP, whether the review should be done by all reviewers or by primary reviewer(s),. In each case a brief summary of the project with informed consent and patient information sheet, advertisements or brochures, if any, should be circulated to all the other members.

**The ethical review should be done in formal meetings and EC should not take decisions through circulation of proposals.** The committee should meet at regular intervals and should not keep a decision pending for more than 3 - 6 months, which may be defined in the SOP.

**Periodic Review:** The ongoing research may be reviewed at regular intervals of six months to one year as may be specified in the SOP of the ethics committee.

**Continuing Review:** The IEC has the responsibility to continue reviewing approved projects for continuation, new information, adverse event monitoring, follow-up and later after completion if need be.

**Interim Review:** Each IEC should decide the special circumstances and the mechanism when an interim review can be resorted to by a sub-committee instead of waiting for the scheduled time of the meeting like re-examination of a proposal already examined by the IEC or any other matter which should be brought to the attention of the IEC. However, decisions taken should be brought to the notice of the main committee.

**Monitoring:** Once IEC gives a certificate of approval, it is the duty of the IEC to monitor the approved studies, therefore an oversight mechanism should be in place. Actual site visits can be made especially in the event of reporting of adverse events or violations of human rights.

Additionally, periodic status reports must be asked for at appropriate intervals based on the safety concerns and this should be specified in the SOP of the IEC. SAE reports from the site as well as other sites are reviewed by EC and appropriate action must be taken when required. In case the IEC desires so, reports of monitoring done by the sponsor and the recommendations of the DSMB may also be sought.

**Special Considerations:** While all the above requirements are applicable to biomedical research as a whole irrespective of the specialty of the research, there are certain specific concerns pertaining to specialised areas of research which require additional safe guards/protection and specific considerations for the IEC to take note of. Examples of such instances are research involving children, pregnant and lactating women, vulnerable participants and those with diminished autonomy besides issues pertaining to commercialisation of research and international collaboration. The observations and suggestions of IEC should be given in writing in unambiguous terms in such instances.

### *ICH Ethical Guidelines Basic Principles* [E6]:

1. The clinical trials should be conducted in accordance with ethical principles which must have their origin to the Declaration of Helsinki.

2. Before a trial is initiated, foreseeable risks and inconvenience should be weighed against the anticipated benefits for the individual trial subject and society.

3. The trials, safety, and well – beings of the trial subjects are the most important consideration and should prevail over interest of science and society.

4. The available non-clinical and clinical information on an investigational product should be adequate to support the proposed clinical trial.

5. Clinical trials should be scientifically sound and described clearly in protocol.

6. A trial should be conducted in compliance with the protocol that has received prior approval from the ethics committee.

7. The medical care given or medical care decisions made for the trail subjects should be the responsibility of a qualified physician or dentist as appropriate.

8. Each individual involved in conducting a trial should be qualified by education, training and experience to perform the tasks.

9. Freely given informed consent should be obtained from every trial subject prior to participation.

10. All clinical trial information should be recorded, handled and stored in a way that allows its accurate reporting, interpretation and verification.

11. The confidentiality of records that could identify subjects should be protected respecting the privacy and confidentiality rules as applicable.

12. The investigational products should be manufactured, handled, and stored in accordance with applicable GMP.

13. Systems with procedures that assure the quality of every aspect of the trial should be implemented.

## General Ethical Issues

All the research involving human participants should be conducted in accordance with the four basic ethical principles: autonomy (respect for person/participant), beneficence, non-maleficence (do no harm) and justice. The guidelines laid down are directed at application of these basic principles to research involving human participants.

The Principal Investigator is the person responsible for not only undertaking research but also for observance of the rights, health and welfare of the participants recruited for the study. S/he should have qualification and competence in biomedical research methodology for proper conduct of the study and should be aware of and comply with the scientific, legal and ethical requirements of the study protocol.

### I. Informed Consent Process

1. **Informed Consent of Participants:** For all biomedical research involving human participants, the investigator must obtain the informed consent of the prospective participant or in the case of an individual who is not capable of giving informed consent, the consent of a legal guardian. **The ethics of informed consent has five elements:**

   - Disclosure of information – The research participants has the right to the information necessary to make his/her decisions and to be informed of the consequences of his/her decision.

   - Comprehension – The participant should understand the purpose of the study. The implications of the participation and implications of not having the test or treatment.

   - Voluntariness (freedom from control by others) – The participant has the right to self-determination.

   - Competence – A mentally competent adult person has the right to give or withhold consent for any procedure.

   - Choice – The children may be able to give consent to some procedures, but not to other complex procedures.

   Adequate information about the research is given in a simple and easily understandable unambiguous language in a document known as the Informed Consent Form (ICF) with Participant/ Patient Information Sheet. The latter should have following components:

   1. Nature and purpose of study stating it as research

2. Duration of participation with number of participants
3. Procedures to be followed
4. Investigations, if any, to be performed
5. Foreseeable risks and discomforts adequately described and whether project involves more than minimal risk
6. Benefits to participant, community or medical profession as may be applicable
7. Policy on compensation
8. Availability of medical treatment for such injuries or risk management
9. Alternative treatments if available
10. Steps taken for ensuring confidentiality
11. No loss of benefits on withdrawal
12. Benefit sharing in the event of commercialization
13. Contact details of PI or local PI/Co-PI in multicentric studies for asking more information related to the research or in case of injury
14. Contact details of Chairman of the IEC for appeal against violation of rights
15. Voluntary participation
16. If test for genetics and HIV is to be done, counselling for consent for testing must be given as per national guidelines
17. Storage period of biological sample and related data with choice offered to participant regarding future use of sample, refusal for storage and receipt of its results

A copy of the participant/patient information sheet should be given to the participant for her/ his record. The informed consent should be brief in content highlighting that it is given of free will or voluntarily after understanding the implications of risks and benefits and s/he could withdraw without loss of routine care benefits.

Assurance is given that confidentiality would be maintained and all the investigations/ interventions would be carried out only after consent is obtained. When the written consent as signature or thumb impression is not possible due to sensitive nature of the project or the participant is unable to write, then verbal consent can be taken after ensuring its documentation by an unrelated witness.

In some cases, ombudsman, a third party, can ensure total accountability for the process of obtaining the consent. Audio-visual methods could be adopted with prior consent and adequate precaution to ensure confidentiality, but approval of EC is required for such procedures. For drug trials, if the volunteer can give only thumb impression, then another thumb impression by the relative or legal custodian cannot be accepted and an unrelated witness to the project should then sign.

**Fresh or re-consent is taken in following conditions:**

1. Availability of new information which would necessitate deviation of protocol.

2. When a research participant regains consciousness from unconscious state or is mentally competent to understand the study. If such an event is expected then procedures to address it should be spelt out in the informed consent form.

3. When long term follow-up or study extension is planned later.

4. When there is a change in treatment modality, procedures, site visits.

5. Before publication, if there is possibility of disclosure of identity through data presentation or photographs (which should be camouflaged adequately).

**Waiver of Consent**

Voluntary informed consent is always a requirement for every research proposal. However, this can be waived if it is justified that the research involves not more than minimal risk or when the participant and the researcher do not come into contact or when it is necessitated in emergency situations. If such studies have protections in place for both privacy and confidentiality, and do not violate the rights of the participants then IECs may waive off the requirement of informed consent in following instances:

(i) When it is impractical to conduct research since confidentiality of personally identifiable information has to be maintained throughout research as may be required by the sensitivity of the research objective, *eg.*, study on disease burden of HIV/AIDS.

(ii) Research on publicly available information, documents, records, works, performances, reviews, quality assurance studies, archival materials or third party interviews, service programs for benefit of public having a bearing on public health programs, and consumer acceptance studies.

  (iii) Research on anonymised biological samples from deceased individuals, left over samples after clinical investigation, cell lines or cell free derivatives like viral isolates, DNA or RNA from recognised institutions or qualified investigators, samples or data from repositories or registries *etc.*

  (iv) In emergency situations when no surrogate consent can be taken.

2. **Obligations of investigators regarding informed consent:** The investigator has the duty to:

  (i) Communicate to the prospective participants on all the information necessary for informed consent. Any restriction on participant's right to ask any questions related to the study will undermine the validity of informed consent;

  (ii) Exclude the possibility of unjustified deception, undue influence and intimidation. Although deception is not permissible, if sometimes such information would jeopardize the validity of research it can be withheld till the completion of the project, for instance, study on abortion practices;

  (iii) Seek consent only after the prospective participant is adequately informed. The investigator should not give any unjustifiable assurances to prospective participant, which may influence her/his decision to participate;

  (iv) Obtain from each prospective participant a signed form as an evidence of informed consent (written informed consent) preferably witnessed by a person not related to the trial, and in case the participant is not competent to do so, a legal guardian or other duly authorised representative;

  (v) Take verbal consent when the participant refuses to sign or give thumb impression or cannot do so. This can then be documented through audio or video means;

  (vi) Take surrogate consent from the authorized relative or legal custodian or the institutional head in case of abandoned institutionalized individuals or wards under judicial custody;

  (vii) Renew or take fresh informed consent of each participant if required;

(viii) Obtain surrogate consent from the authorized person or legal custodian if participant loses consciousness or competence to consent during the research period as in Alzeimer or psychiatric conditions,

(ix) Assure prospective participants that their decision to participate or not will not affect the patient - clinician relationship or any other benefits to which they are entitled.

3. **Essential information for prospective research participants:** The investigator must provide the individual with the following information in an understandable language by the prospective participant before seeking an individual's consent to participate in research:

(i) The aims and methods of the research;

(ii) The expected duration of the participation;

(iii) The benefits that might reasonably be expected as an outcome of research to the participant or community or to others;

(iv) Any alternative procedures or courses of treatment that might be as advantageous to the participant as the procedure or treatment to which s/he is being subjected;

(v) Any foreseeable risk or discomfort to the participant resulting from participation in the study;

(vi) Right to prevent use of her/ his biological sample (DNA, cell-line, etc.) at any time during the course of the research;

(vii) The extent to which confidentiality of records could be maintained i.e., the limits to which the investigator would be able to safeguard confidentiality and the anticipated consequences of breach of confidentiality;

(viii) Responsibility of investigators;

(ix) Free treatment for research related injury by the investigator and/or institution or sponsor;

(x) Compensation for participants for disability or death resulting from such injury;

(xi) Insurance coverage if any, for research related or other AEs;

(xii) Freedom of individual / family to participate and to withdraw from the research any time without penalty or loss of benefits which the participant would otherwise be entitled to;

(xiii) The identity of the research teams and contact persons with address and phone numbers;

(xiv) Foreseeable extent of information on possible current and future uses of the biological material and of the data to be generated from the research and if the material is likely to be used for secondary purposes or would be shared with others, clear mention of the same;

(xv) Risk of discovery of biologically sensitive information and provision to safeguard confidentiality;

(xvi) Publications, if any, including photographs and pedigree charts. The quality of the consent of certain social and marginalized groups requires careful consideration as their agreement to volunteer may be unduly influenced by the Investigator.

The information given must not only be scientifically accurate but should also be sensitive/ adaptive to their social and cultural context.

## II. Compensation for Participation

The participants may be paid for the inconvenience and time spent, and should be reimbursed for expenses incurred, in connection with their participation in the research. They may also receive free medical services. When this is reasonable then it cannot be termed as benefit.

During the period of research if the participant requires treatment for complaints other than the one being studied necessary, free ancillary care or appropriate referrals may be provided. However, payments should not be so large or the medical services so extensive as to make prospective participants consent readily to enroll in research against their better judgment, which would then be treated as undue inducement.

All payments, reimbursements and medical services that are to be provided to research participants should be approved by the IEC.

*Care should be taken:*

(i) when a guardian is asked to give consent on behalf of an incompetent person, no remuneration should be offered except a refund of out of pocket expenses;

(ii) when a participant is withdrawn from research for medical reasons related to the study, the participant should get the benefit for full participation;

(iii) when a participant withdraws for any other reasons, s/he should be paid an amount proportionate to the amount of participation.

## III. Conflict of Interest

A set of conditions in which professional judgment concerning a primary interest like patient's welfare or the validity of research tends to be or appears to be unduly influenced by a secondary interest like non-financial (personal, academic or political) or financial gain is termed as Conflict of Interest (COI).

Academic institutions conducting research in alliance with industries/ commercial companies require a strong review to probe possible conflicts of interest between scientific responsibilities of researchers and business interests (ownership or part-ownership of a company developing a new product). In cases where the review board/ committee determines that a conflict of interest may damage the scientific integrity of a project or cause harm to research participants, the board/ committee should advise accordingly.

Significant financial interest means anything of monetary value that would reasonably appear to be a significant consequence of such research including salary or other payments for services like consulting fees or honorarium per participant; equity interests in stocks, stock options or other ownership interests; and intellectual property rights from patents, copyrights and royalties from such rights. The investigators should declare such conflicts of interest in the application submitted to the IEC for review.

Institutions and IECs need self-regulatory processes to monitor, prevent and resolve such conflicts of interest. The IEC can determine the conditions for management of such conflicts in its SOP manual. Prospective participants in research should also be informed of the sponsorship of research, so that they can be aware of the potential for conflicts of interest and commercial aspects of the research. The secondary financial interest is also to be informed while presenting papers or publishing.

Undue inducement through compensation for individual participants, families and populations should be prohibited. This prohibition however, does not include agreements with individuals, families, groups, communities or populations that foresee technology transfer, local training, joint ventures, provision of health care reimbursement, costs of travel and loss of wages and the possible use of a percentage of any royalties for humanitarian purposes. Undue compensation would include assistance to related person(s) for transport of body for cremation or burial, provision for insurance for unrelated conditions, free transportation to and fro for examination not included in the routine, free trip to town if the participants are from rural areas, free hot meals, freedom for prisoners, free medication which is generally not available, academic credits and disproportionate compensation to researcher / team/ institution. However, in remote and inaccessible areas some of the features mentioned above may be a necessity and culture specific. Therefore, the IEC should examine this on a case-by-case basis, as some of these elements may be justifiable for collecting vital data for national use or necessary to find if some interventions may significantly have direct impact on health policies.

**IV. Selection of Special Groups as Research Participants**

1. **Pregnant or nursing women:** Pregnant or nursing women should in no circumstances be the participant of any research unless the research carries    no more than minimal risk to the fetus or nursing infant and the object of the research is to obtain new knowledge about the foetus, pregnancy and lactation.

   As a general rule, pregnant or nursing women should not be participants of any clinical trial except such trials as are designed to protect or advance the    health of pregnant or nursing women or foetuses or nursing infants, and for which the women who are not pregnant or nursing would not be suitable participants.

   (a) The justification of participation of these women in clinical trials would be that they should not be deprived arbitrarily of the opportunity to benefit from investigations, drugs, vaccines or other agents that promise therapeutic or preventive benefits. Example of such trials is, to test the efficacy and safety of a drug for reducing prenatal transmission of HIV infection from mother to child, trials for detecting foetal abnormalities and for conditions associated with or aggravated by pregnancy etc. Women should not be encouraged to discontinue nursing for the sake of participation in research and in case she decides to do so, harm of cessation of breast-feeding to the nursing child should be properly assessed except in those studies where breast feeding is harmful to the infant. Compensation in terms of supplying supplementary food such as milk formula should be considered in such instances.

(b) Research related to termination of pregnancy: Pregnant women who desire to undergo Medical Termination of Pregnancy (MTP) could be made participants for such research as per The Medical Termination of Pregnancy Act, GOI, 1971.

(c) Research related to pre-natal diagnostic techniques: In pregnant women such research should be limited to detect the foetal abnormalities or genetic disorders as per the Prenatal Diagnostic Techniques (Regulation and Prevention of Misuse) Act, GOI, 1994 and not for sex determination of the foetus.

2. **Children:** Before undertaking trial in children the investigator must ensure that

(a) Children will not be involved in research that could be carried out equally well with adults;

(b) The purpose of the research is to obtain knowledge relevant to health needs of children. For clinical evaluation of a new drug the study in children should always be carried out after the phase III clinical trials in adults. It can be studied earlier only if the drug has a therapeutic value in a primary disease of the children;

(c) A parent or legal guardian of each child has given proxy consent;

(d) The assent of the child should be obtained to the extent of the child's capabilities such as in the case of mature minors from the age of seven years up to the age of 18 years;

(e) Research should be conducted in settings where the child and parent can obtain adequate medical and psychological support;

(f) Interventions intended to provide direct diagnostic, therapeutic or preventive benefit for the individual child participant must be justified in relation to anticipated risks involved in the study and anticipated benefits to society;

(g) The child's refusal to participate in research must always be respected unless there is no medically acceptable alternative to the therapy provided/ tested, provided the consent has been obtained from parents / guardian;

(h) Interventions that are intended to provide therapeutic benefit are likely to be atleast as advantageous to the individual child participant as any available alternative interventions;

(i) The risk presented by interventions not intended to benefit the individual child participant is low when compared to the importance of the knowledge that is to be gained.

Article 12 of the United Nations Convention on the Rights of the Child (1989) states: "A child who is capable of forming his/her views has the right to express these views freely on all matters affecting the child, the views of the child being given due weight in accordance of the age and maturity of the child".

3. **Vulnerable groups:** Effort may be made to ensure that individuals or communities invited for research be selected in such a way that the burdens and benefits of the research are equally distributed.

   (a) Research on genetics should not lead to racial inequalities;

   (b) Persons who are economically or socially disadvantaged should not be used to benefit those who are better off than them;

   (c) Rights and welfare of mentally challenged and mentally differently able persons who are incapable of giving informed consent or those with behavioral disorders must be protected. Appropriate proxy consent from the legal guardian should be taken after the person is well informed about the study, need for participation, risks and benefits involved and the privacy and confidentiality procedures. The entire consent process should be properly documented;

   (d) Adequate justification is required for the involvement of participants such as prisoners, students, subordinates, employees, service personnel etc., who have reduced autonomy as research participants, since the consent provided may be under duress or various other compelling reasons.

## V. Essential Information on Confidentiality for Prospective Research Participants

***Safeguarding confidentiality:*** The investigator must safeguard the confidentiality of research data, which might lead to the identification of the individual participants.

Data of individual participants can be disclosed under the following circumstances:

(a) only in a court of law under the orders of the presiding judge; or

(b) there is threat to a person's life; or

(c) in cases of severe adverse reactions which may be required to communicate to drug registration authority; or

(d) if there is risk to public health it takes precedence over personal right to privacy and may have to be communicated to health authority.

Therefore, the limitations in maintaining the confidentiality of data should be anticipated and assessed and communicated to appropriate individuals or authorities as the case may be.

## VI. Compensation for Accidental Injury

Research participants who suffer physical injury as a result of their participation are entitled to financial or other assistance to compensate them equitably for any temporary or permanent impairment or disability. In case of death, their dependents are entitled to material compensation. The DCGI now made the CROs responsible for compensating clinical trial injuries by including a new clause in trial approval letters.

***Obligation of the sponsor to pay:*** The sponsor whether a pharmaceutical company, a government, or an institution, should agree, before the research begins, in the *a priori* agreement to provide compensation for any physical or psychological injury for which participants are entitled or agree to provide insurance coverage for an unforeseen injury whenever possible.

An Arbitration committee or appellate authority could be set up by the institution to decide on the issue of compensation on a case-by-case basis for larger trials. Alternately an institution can also establish such a committee to oversee such claims, which would be common for projects being undertaken by it.

Compensation for ancillary care for unrelated illness as free treatment or appropriate referrals may also be included in the *a priori* agreement with the sponsors whenever possible.

## VII. Post - Trial Access

It is necessary during the study planning process to identify post-trial access by study participants to prophylactic, diagnostic and therapeutic procedures identified as beneficial in the study or access to other appropriate care. Post-trial access arrangements or other care must be described in the study protocol so that ethical review committee may consider such arrangements during its review.

The IEC should consider such an arrangement in the *priori* agreement. Sometimes more than the benefit to the participant, the community may be given benefit in indirect way through improving their living conditions, establishing counseling centers, clinics or schools, and giving education on maintaining good health practices. For smaller scale or student projects post trial benefit to the participants may not be feasible but keeping in mind the post trial responsibility, conscious efforts should be made by the guides and the institution to initiate steps to continue to support and give better care to the participants.

## VIII. International Collaboration / Assistance in Bio-Medical / Health Research

On one hand the collaboration in medical research suggests an interest in a humane and civil society while on the other it could give the impression of experimentation on the population of one country by another. Different levels of development in terms of infrastructure, expertise, social and cultural perceptions, laws relating to intellectual property rights etc., necessitate an ethical framework to guide such collaboration. The same concerns are applicable even when there is no formal collaboration between countries, but the research is undertaken with assistance from international organisations as sponsors (Governmental bodies like National Institutes of Health, USA, non-Government bodies like Bill & Melinda Gates Foundation, Ford Foundation or others like WHO, UNICEF, UNAIDS, etc.).

### Special Concerns

1. Given the magnitude and severity of the health problems in different countries, capacity building to address ethical issues

that arise out of collaborative research must be promoted on a priority basis. Strategies should be implemented so that various countries and communities can practice meaningful self-determination in health development and can ensure the scientific and ethical conduct of research.

2. The collaborating investigators, institutions and countries can function as equal partners with sponsors even when in a vulnerable position by building appropriate safeguards. Community representatives should be involved early enough while designing the protocol and in a sustained manner during the development, implementation, monitoring and dissemination of results of research.

3. Careful consideration should be given to protect the dignity, safety and welfare of the participants when the social contexts of the proposed research can create foreseeable conditions for exploitation of the participants or increase their vulnerability to harm. The steps to be taken to overcome these should be described and approval taken from concerned IEC/IndEC.

4. Every adult participant in the research should voluntarily give informed consent and also that of child as may be applicable.

5. As different kinds of research (epidemiological studies, clinical trials, product development, behavioural and social science oriented research *etc.*) have their own particular scientific requirements and specific ethical challenges, the choice of study populations for each type of study should be justified in advance in scientific and ethical terms regardless of the place from where the study population is selected. Generally, early clinical phases of research, particularly of drugs, vaccines and devices, should be conducted in communities that are less vulnerable to harm or exploitation. However, for valid scientific and public health reasons, if sufficient scientific and ethical safeguards are ensured it may be conducted in any place after obtaining relevant regulatory clearances.

6. The nature, magnitude, and probability of all foreseeable harms resulting from participation in a collaborative research programme should be specified in the research protocol and explained to the participants as fully as can be reasonably done. Moreover, the modalities by which to address these, including provision for the best possible nationally available care to

participants who experience adverse reactions to a vaccine or drug under study, compensation for injury related to the research, and referral for psychosocial and legal support if necessary, need to be described.

7. The research protocol should outline the benefits that persons / communities / countries participating in such research should experience as a result of their participation. Care should be taken so that these are not presented in a way that unduly influences freedom of choice in participation. The burden and the benefit should be equally borne by the collaborating countries.

8. Guidelines, rules, regulations and cultural sensitivities of all countries participating in collaborative research projects should be respected, especially by researchers in the host country and the sponsor country. These could be with reference to intellectual property rights, exchange of biological materials (human, animal, plant or microbial), data transfer, security issues, and issues of socially or politically sensitive nature. In this context, it is essential for researchers to follow the GOI notification on "Exchange of Human Biological Material for Biomedical Research" issued on 19.11.97 and obtain appropriate regulatory clearances as prevalent in the country for international collaboration and EC approval from all trial sites before the initiation of research.

## IX. Researcher's Relations with the Media and Publication Practices

The researchers have a responsibility to make sure that the public is accurately informed about the results without raising false hopes or expectations. It should also not unnecessarily scare the people. Researchers should take care to avoid talking with journalists or reporters about preliminary findings as seemingly promising research that subsequently cannot be validated or could lead to misconcepts if reported prematurely.

Or, the results of research may be reported in such a way that it would seem that the human application is round the corner, only to be told later by the researchers that considerable time has to pass before these findings can be translated into tools for human use. In such circumstances, retractions most often do not appear in the media. Therefore, it is important to avoid premature reports and publicity stunts. The best safeguard against inaccurate reporting is for the researcher to talk to media on condition that the reporter submit a full written, rather than oral version, of what will be reported, so that it enables the researcher to make necessary corrections, if needed, prior to publication.

Investigator's publication plans should not threaten the privacy or confidentiality of participants, for example publication of pedigrees in the report on research in genetics can result in identification of study participants. It is recommended that a clear consent for publication be obtained besides the consent for participation in research or treatment and such a consent should preferably be obtained on two different occasions and not as a blanket one at the commencement of the study. Maintenance of confidentiality while publishing data should be taken care of. In case there is need for publication / presentation of photographs/ slides / videos of participant (s), prior consent to do so should be obtained. Identification features should be appropriately camouflaged. The same safeguard should be observed for video coverage.

Only those who make substantial contribution to the article and take responsibility for the published matter can be co-authors. Plagiarism or falsification of data and authorship are important ethical issues in publications. The term 'misconduct in research' means fabrication, falsification, plagiarism, selective omission of data and claiming that some data are missing, ignoring outliers without declaring it, not reporting data on side effects/ adverse reactions in a clinical trial, publication of post-hoc analysis without declaring it, gift authorship, not citing others' work, not disclosing conflict of interest, redundant publication, and failure to adequately review existing research.

## Specific Principles for Drug Trials

The clinical trial should be carried out only after approval of the Drugs Controller General of India (DCGI) as is necessary under the Schedule 'Y' of Drugs and Cosmetics Rules 1945 (Drugs and Cosmetics Act 1940). The investigator should also get the approval of the Ethical Committee of the Institution before submitting the proposal to DCGI. All the guiding principles should be followed irrespective of whether the drug has been developed in this country or abroad or whether clinical trials have been carried out outside India or not.

Throughout the drug trials, the distinction between therapy and research should be maintained. A physician /investigator who participates in research by administering the new drug to consenting patients should ensure that the patients understand and remember that the drug is experimental and that its benefits for the condition under study are yet unproven.

The clinical trial of drugs is a randomized single or double blind controlled study in human participants, designed to evaluate prospectively the safety and effectiveness of new drugs/ new formulations.

***Special considerations***

(i)   Use of a placebo in drug trials and sham surgery has been intensely debated (Current version of Helsinki Declaration (2008) discourages the use of placebo). Each protocol using placebo requires careful consideration before approval. Denial of the available treatment to control (placebo) group of patients is unethical.

(ii)  Trials of drugs without the approval of the Indian Regulatory Authority and appropriate agencies should be dealt according to the law of the land.

(iii) After the clinical trial is over, if the drug is found effective, it should be made mandatory that the sponsoring agency should provide the drug to the patient till it is marketed in the country and thereafter at a reduced rate for the participants whenever possible. A suitable *a priori* agreement should be reached on post trial benefits.

(iv)  The criteria for termination of a trial must be defined *a priori* in the proposal of the trial and plan of interim analysis must be clearly presented. This is important when on interim analysis the test drug is found to be clearly more effective or less effective than the standard drug. The trial can be discontinued thereafter and better drug should be given to patient receiving less effective drug.

(v)   Issues of partner notification and discordant couples should be taken care of before initiating any HIV/ AIDS related trial.

(vi)  For new drug substances discovered in India, clinical trials are required to be carried out in India right from Phase I through Phase III and data should be submitted as required specified in Schedule 'Y' of Drugs and Cosmetics Rules. Permission to carry out these trials shall generally be given in stages, considering the data emerging from earlier Phase(s).

(vii) For new drug substances discovered in countries other than India, Phase I data from other country(ies) should be submitted along with the application. After Phase I data generated outside India has been submitted to the Licensing Authority, permission may be granted to conduct Phase II and Phase III trials concurrently with other global trials for that drug.

(viii) In case of amendment or deviation in the protocol not only the approval of IEC may be obtained but also the Licensing Authority is to be notified of the same. In order to optimize and expedite drug development for drugs indicated in life threatening/ serious diseases or specific diseases of relevance to India – the toxicological and clinical data requirements shall be decided on a case by case basis. In such cases, particular studies may be abbreviated, deferred or omitted, as deemed appropriate by the Licensing Authority and not by ECs.

The Indian Good Clinical Practices (GCP) provide operative guidelines for ethical and scientific standards for the designing of a trial protocol including conduct, recording and reporting procedures and should be strictly adhered to while carrying out a trial.

***Some International Unethical Human Experimentations:***
1. *Nazi Experiment:* During the Second World War the Nazi Physicians committed innumerable atrocities on uninformed prisoners of war in the name of medical research. Some of the so called experiments include: high altitude experiments, freezing experiments, malaria and typhus experiments, sulphanilamide and poison experiments, phosphorous burns and chemical sterilization. Besides these, hundreds of prisoners were killed to collect skeletons for an anthropological investigation. This came to the light during the Nuremberg Military Tribunal's meeting which shocked the entire world. In addition to sentencing the accused, the Military Tribunal Judges articulated the Nuremberg Code in 1947. This is the new beginning in ethics for medical research. The code outlined 10 principles which need to be observed during research to satisfy moral, ethical and legal concepts.

- Freezing Experiments: were conducted on men to simulate the conditions the armies suffered on the Eastern Front. The German forces were ill prepared for the bitter cold. The freezing experiments were divided into two parts. First, to establish how long it would take to lower the body temperature to death and second how to best resuscitate the frozen victim. The two main methods used to freeze the victim were to put the person in a icy vat of water or to put the victim outside naked in sub-zero temperatures. They were usually stripped naked and prepared for the experiment. An insulated probe which measured the drop in the body temperature was inserted into the rectum. The probe was held in place by a expandable metal ring which was adjusted to open inside the rectum to hold the probe firmly in place. The victim was then placed in the vat of cold water and started to freeze. It was learned that most victims lost consciousness and died when the body temperature dropped to –25 °C.

- Sulphonamide Experiments: Wounds inflicted on the subjects were infected with bacteria such as *Streptococcus, Clostridium perfringens and Clostridium tetani.* Circulation of blood was interrupted by tying off blood vessels at both ends of the wound to create a condition similar to that of a battlefield wound. Infection was aggravated by forcing wood shavings and ground glass into the wounds. The infection was treated with sulfonamide and other drugs to determine their effectiveness.

2. *Tuskegee Syphilis Study:* This study was conducted in Alabama county in which more than 400 African Americans were observed for natural history of syphilis without any intervention although penicillin had been discovered and found to be a cure for syphilis. They were not informed about the true nature of the study and were followed for 40 years until exposed by a press reporter in 1972. The study exemplified a pattern of institutionalized racism in health care and ultimately after 25 years of enquiry President Bill Clinton of USA in 1997 tendered a public apology and paid as compensation 7 billion US Dollars in addition to setting up of the Tuskegee University National Centre for Bioethics in Research and Health. This study led to the release of first ever National Guidelines, known as Belmont Report, in 1979.

### *Some Indian Unethical Human Experimentations:*

Recent times have witnessed a number of exposes and scandals in clinical trials and it is expected that quietly there may be a lot more happening in the country.

1. Trial of a New Pneumonia Vaccine (2008): A Hyderabad based CRO was conducting trial of new pneumonia vaccine on behalf of US based pharmaceutical company in private medical college hospital at Bangalore. An infant is reported to have died after being administered the trial vaccine. For the first time the regulatory authority (DCGI) investigated the issue which revealed that infant had a heart condition. The trial had been meant to be conducted on healthy babies. The investigation further revealed that the informed consent was not taken before the vaccine was administered. The medical college hospital's ethics committee was not properly constituted as it was not chaired by an external member to ensure independent functioning.

   (*Sandhya Srinivasan* Bodies for hire; The outsourcing of clinical trials **August 2009**)

2. Bioequivalence Study of Felodipine: In December 2008, a person is reported to have died in a bioequivalence study of a blood pressure drug felodipine. Such study is conducted in healthy volunteers. The Hyderabad based CRO who was conducting the study reported that the person had been taking part in multiple trial which could have accounted for his death. If the person had taken part in many trials, it would only have been for the money, which would amount to an inducement according to national and international ethical guidelines for research – an inducement that might have made him overlook the risks of the trials. And, in any case, why did the company let him take part in the felodipine trial when it was aware that he had taken part in many others?

   (*Sandhya Srinivasan* Bodies for hire; The outsourcing of clinical trials **August 2009**)

3. Experimental Stent (2006): A Dutch Medical Equipment producer had tested an experimental stent on about 70 Indian heart patients without telling them that this was the part of the test. Neither had there been approval from ethical review committee.

   The special stent was later introduced in Dutch market. The stent was meant to open congested coronary arteries and also to deliver medicines. It was alleged that a deliberate decision had been made not to ask for permission in order to circumvent the complicated and time consuming ethical procedures that surround clinical trials. A number of patients who had assumed that they were receiving conventional treatment are now demanding compensation for having been used as guinea pigs without their knowledge and also for having had to pay a large sum of money to have the stent implanted, despite the fact that such payments are explicitly forbidden by regulators.

This was exposed in a Dutch documentary television programme which showed all evidence. But the Dutch company as well as Indian hospital denied carrying out such trial.

(A Bitter Pill – WEMOS, December 2007)

**Example of an Informed Consent Form**

**(Source: Workbook for Investigators, TDR/PRD/GCP/02.1B, 2002)**

The doctor has confirmed that you have the skin disease called salak. As you probably know, this disease is very common in this area, and is transmitted by the bite of a sandfly. If not treated, your sore will probably increase in size and cause a lot of discomfort to you, but after sometime they may heal by themselves, producing deep scars. Unfortunately, the medicines available for treatment are not very good – several injections are required, and you may experience vomiting and pain at the site of injection.

The Centre for Research and Training in Skin Diseases and leprosy is looking for better drugs that can be given by mouth, and a cream that can be applied to the sores. From the experience we have had with the treatment of other skin diseases using medicines called fluconazole and a cream that contains a drug called ketoconazole, we believe that this may also be a good treatment for salak.

The Centre is now inviting (recruiting) around 200 patients with salak to participate in a study to see whether this new treatment can be used to cure salak. If you agree to participate in the study, we will provide you all the explanation you need, and you will receive special medical attention from the centre.

In order to see if this medication really is good for salak, we need to compare the results of treatment with results from another group of patients who will receive some pills and a cream which look similar but have no effect on sores. The doctors will examine each patient several times during the course of treatment. Neither the doctors nor the patients will know which medication and cream was given.

The treatment will be provided to you at no cost. It will consist of taking one pill a day and applying the cream twice a day. Depending on the type of disease you have, the treatment may last for a period of 6 or 12 weeks. You will have to come back here 3, 6 and 12 weeks after starting treatment to collect the medication , see the doctor, and have some laboratory tests done. Each time, the laboratory technician will prepare a slide from a scrapping of your sores.

The Centre will compensate you if you have to leave your work to come here, and will pay for transportation between your home and centre. We are going to pay careful attention, in case the medication has any undesired effect on you, and a blood examination will be performed when you finish the treatment after 3 weeks or after 6 and 12 weeks if you have to be treated for 12 weeks.

Only patients in good health will be invited to participate, and an initial blood test will be carried out to check your condition of health. The total amount of blood collected for examination each time will not be more than a regular syringe (10 ml) full. You should know that this new treatment may produce, in more sensitive patients, some vomiting and skin rash.  If you feel any discomfort, please come to the Centre at any time. The doctor will decide if you can continue the medication or should withdraw from the trial for safety reasons and be treated with an alternative drug. The centre will be responsible for any additional treatment you may need as a consequence of this disease or the new treatment.

You are not obliged to enter into this study, and in this case the standard injectable medication will be offered to you, consisting of ---- injections of glucantine. On the other hand, if you agree to participate, we would very much like you to follow all the medical instructions, but you should know that you can leave the study at any time without any prejudice of healthcare in the future for you and your family.

All the information collected from you during the trial will be kept confidential. If the results of the trial are published, your identity will remain confidential.

This study has been approved by the Ministry of Health and Tehran University, which gave the approval on ------.

If you have any further questions, you can contact a member of staff at the clinic of Dr. -------Address----------------------Phone number----------.

If any relevant information which would modify your participation in the trial should become available during the course of treatment, you will be informed by the physician.

In case of any urgency regarding the treatment, you can contact Dr. --------- at any time through his/her private telephone number ----------------------- home address ----------------------

**Consent From**

I have read the information in this form, or it has been read to me. I have had the opportunity to ask questions about it and any questions that I have asked have been answered to my satisfaction. I know that I can refuse to participate in the study without penalty or the loss of benefit to which I have been otherwise entitled or services to which I or my family are entitled.

I freely agree to participate in the study. After signing below, I shall receive a copy of this consent form.

By signing this form I agree that the data collected about me will be accessible to sponsor's representatives (monitors/auditors/--), ethics committee and the regulatory authorities.

PRINT NAME OF PARTICIPANT            DATE AND SIGNATURE

------------------------------------------            -----/-----/-------- (dd/mm/yy)

Subject inclusion no.--------------------            ------------------------

PRINT NAME OF THE WITNESS            DATE AND SIGNATURE

------------------------------------------            -----/-----/------- (dd/mm/yy)

                                                     ------------------------------------

PRINT NAME OF THE WITNESS            DATE AND SIGNATURE

------------------------------------------            -----/-----/------- (dd/mm/yy)

                                                     ------------------------------------

## Key Points to Remember

- The four basic principles of ethics related to human experimentations are: beneficence, non-maleficence, respect for rights and justice.

- Registration of ethics committee is mandatory since 2013 for reviewing and according approval for clinical trials.

- Helsinki declaration is the backbone of developing ethical guideless worldwide. This discourages the use of placebo in the controlled trials when a treatment exists.

- The ICMR code of ethics has 12 principles which need to be followed while carrying out research on human beings. These are: principles of essentiality; voluntariness, informed consent and community agreements; non exploitation; privacy and confidentiality; precaution and risk minimization; professional competence; accountability and transparency; maximization public interest and of distributive justice; institutional arrangements; public domain; totality of responsibility; and compliance.

- Responsibilities of Ethics Committee:
  o The prime responsibility is to safeguard the rights, safety and well-beings of research participants.
  o To function in compliance with regulation and GCP guidance for composition to procedure.
  o It decides on the number of trials per investigator at any time and the site for the clinical trials.
  o To analyze and forward its opinion on serious adverse events to CDSCO.

- **Composition of EC:** minimum of seven members and the chairman must be from outside the institution. Other members should be from scientific, non-scientific, medical and non-medical discipline including one lay public. The medical scientists and clinicians must be post graduates.

- **Review:** For review of each protocol, the quorum of ethics committee should have at least 5 members consisting of basic medical scientist, clinician, legal expert, social scientist, and lay person.

- EC should have its own SOP on functioning with the components like objectives, role, composition, authority for constitution, membership requirements, quorum requirements, offices, provision of consultants, application submission procedure, documentation, review procedure, elements of review, expedite / interim review, decision making, communicating the decision, follow up procedures, archiving and record keeping, and updating EC members.

- All records of EC are to be preserved for at least 5 years from the date of completion or suspension of trials.

- The ethics of consent has five components: disclosure of information, comprehension, voluntariness, competence and choice.

- Information consent form should have the following components: Nature and purpose of study stating it as research; Duration of participation with number of participants; Procedures to be followed; Investigations, if any, to be performed; Foreseeable risks and discomforts adequately described and whether project involves more than minimal risk; Benefits to participant, community or medical profession as may be applicable; Policy on compensation; Availability of medical treatment for such injuries or risk management; Alternative treatments if available; Steps taken for ensuring confidentiality; No loss of benefits on withdrawal; Benefit sharing in the event of commercialization; Contact details of PI or local PI/Co-PI in multi-centric studies for asking more information related to the research or in case of injury; Contact details of Chairman of the IEC for appeal against violation of rights; Voluntary participation; If test for genetics and HIV is to be done, counselling for consent for testing must be given as per national guidelines; Storage period of biological sample and related data with choice offered to participant regarding future use of sample, refusal for storage and receipt of its results.

# CHAPTER 6

# Good Clinical (Research) Practices (GCP) for Clinical Research in India

'Research has been called a good business, a necessity, a gamble, a game.
It is none of these. It is a state of mind'

Martin H. Fischer

**After reading this chapter, you should be able to know or learn:**

- The scope of Good Clinical Practice (GCP);

- Genesis of development of GCP in India;

- The responsibilities of all stake holders of clinical research: sponsor, investigators, ethics committees and others;

- The components of a research protocol, basic ethical principles for clinical research, functioning of ethics committees, concept of quality assurance and data management; and

- Special requirements of clinical trials of vaccines, contraceptives, surgical procedures or medical devices, diagnostic agents and herbal medicines.

Good Clinical Research Practices (GCP) is a process that incorporates established ethical and scientific quality standards for the design, conduct, recording and reporting of clinical research involving the participation of human subjects. Compliance of GCP provides public assurance that rights, safety and well being of research participants are protected and respected, and the study is conducted in consistence with legal and ethical requirements.

The responsibility of GCP is shared by all stake holders like sponsors, investigators, site staff, contract research organizations, ethics committee, regulatory authorities and research subjects. Conducting clinical research in accordance with the principles of GCP helps to ensure that the clinical research participants are not exposed to undue risk and that data generated from the research are valid and accurate.

Adopting GCP guidelines require not only a knowledge of them, but also resourcefulness, or the tact to practice them. The readers may find some of the materials described in the chapter are similar with that described in Ethical Issues in Clinical Research chapter.

***Evolution of Indian GCP:*** The revelation of inhuman and barbaric treatment exposed to inmates of concentration camps by the Nazi doctors during World War II caused a wide spread concern all over the globe. This led to the formulation of Nuremberg Code in 1949 and was followed by World Medical Association's Declaration of Helsinki in 1964. The Declaration of Helsinki has been amended several times latest being in 2014. The Declaration of Helsinki forms the basis of various GCP guidelines.

As the whole world has been looking forward to India as their destination for clinical research, the Government of India felt the need to develop our own Indian Guidelines to ensure uniform quality of clinical research throughout the country and to generate data for registration of new drugs before use in the Indian population. An Expert Committee set up by Central Drugs Standard Control Organisation (CDSCO) in consultation with clinical expert has formulated this GCP guideline for generation of clinical data on drugs. The Drug Technical Advisory Board (DTAB), the highest technical body under D&C Act, has endorsed adoption of this GCP guideline for streamlining the clinical studies in India. This guideline was released in 2001 and this GCP is the standard, clinical researchers need to follow and comply. However, in case of international clinical trial, it is necessary to follow the International Conference on Harmonization (ICH) guidelines in addition to GOI's guidelines.

Several GCP guidelines are available. To cite few Indian GCP guideline, WHO GCP guideline, ICH guideline, US-FDA guideline, European GCP guideline. ICH GCP is available in the accompanying CD.

**Evolution of Indian GCP:**

1. Nuremberg Code in1949.
2. Declaration of Helsinki in1964 (revised on several occasions)
3. ICH GCP in1996.
4. ICMR's "Policy Statement on Ethical Considerations for Research on Human Subjects" 1980.
5. The ICMR's guideline "Ethical Guidelines for Biomedical Research on Human Subject" in 2000.
6. GCP Guideline, CDSCO, 2001.
7. Revised Schedule Y to Drugs and Cosmetics Rules, 2005.
8. ICMR's revised "Ethical Guidelines for Biomedical Research on Human Participants, Indian Council of Medical Research", 2006.
9. Mandatory registration of ethics committee – 2013
10. Revision of National Ethical Guidelines – Draft released by ICMR in 2016.

The salient points of Indian GCP are discussed below. It is not intended to completely produce the full GCP. The readers are encouraged to refer the full text if they need.

## Prerequisites for the Study

### Investigational Pharmaceutical Product

Physical, chemical, pharmaceutical properties and the formulation of the Investigational Product must be documented to permit appropriate safety measures to be taken during the course of a study. Instructions for the storage and handling of the dosage form should be documented. Any structural similarity(ies) to the other known compounds should be mentioned.

### Pre-clinical supporting data

The available pre-clinical data and clinical information on the Investigational Product should be adequate and convincing to support the proposed study.

## Protocol

### Relevant components of Protocol

#### *General information*

(a) Protocol title, protocol identifying number and date. All amendments should bear amendment number and date(s)

(b) Name, address & contact numbers of the sponsor and the monitor / CRO

(c) Name and title of the persons authorised to sign the protocol and the protocol amendments for the sponsor

(d) Name, title, address and contact numbers of the sponsor's medical expert for the study

(e) Name(s), title(s), address(es) and contact numbers of the investigator(s) who is / are responsible for conducting the study, along with their consent letter(s)

(f) Name(s), address(es) and contact numbers of the institution(s) - clinical laboratories and / or other medical and technical departments along with the particulars of the head(s) of the institution(s) and the relevant department(s)

#### *Objectives and Justification*

(a) Aims and objectives of the study, indicating the phase to which the study corresponds

(b) Name and description of the investigational product(s)

(c) A summary of findings from non-clinical studies that potentially have clinical significance and from clinical studies those are relevant to the study

(d) Summary of the known and potential risks and benefits, if any, to human subjects

(e) Description of and justification for the route of administration, dosage regimen and treatment periods for the pharmaceutical product being studied and the product being used as control. Dose-response relationships should be considered and stated.

(f) A statement that the study will be conducted in compliance with the protocol, GCP and the applicable regulatory requirements

(g) Description of the inclusion & exclusion criteria of the study population

(h) References to the literature and data that are relevant to the study and that provide background for the study

### *Ethical Considerations*

(a) General ethical considerations related to the study

(b) Description of how patients / healthy volunteers will be informed and how their consent will be obtained

(c) Possible reasons for not seeking informed consent

## *Study design*

The scientific integrity of the study and the credibility of the data from the study depend substantially on the study design. Description of the study design should include:

(a) Specific statement of primary and secondary end points, if any, to be measured during the study

(b) Description of the type of the study (randomised, comparative, blinded, open, placebo controlled), study design (parallel groups, cross-over technique), blinding technique (double-blind, single-blind), randomisation (method and procedure) and placebo controlled.

(c) A schematic diagram of the study design, procedures and stages

(d) Medications/treatments permitted (including rescue medications) and not permitted before and / or during the study

(e) A description of the study treatments, dosage regimen, route of administration and the dosage form of the investigational product and the control proposed during the study

(f) A description of the packaging and labelling of the investigational product

(g) Duration of the subject participation and a description of the sequence of all study periods including follow-up, if any

(h) Proposed date of initiation of the study

(i) Justification of the time-schedules e.g. in the light of how far the safety of the active ingredients, medicinal products has been tested, the time course of the disease in question

(j) Discontinuation criteria for study subjects and instructions on terminating or suspending the whole study or a part of the study

(k) Accountability procedures for the investigational products including the comparator product

(l) Maintenance of study treatment randomisation codes and procedures for breaking codes

(m) Documentation of any decoding that may occur during the study

(n) Procedures for monitoring subjects' compliance

### *Inclusion, Exclusion and Withdrawal of Subjects*

(a) Subject inclusion criteria: specifications of the subjects (patients / healthy volunteers) including age, gender, ethnic groups, prognostic factors, diagnostic admission criteria etc. should be clearly mentioned where relevant.

(b) Subject exclusion criteria, including an exhaustive statement on the criteria for pre-admission exclusions

(c) Subject withdrawal criteria (i.e. terminating investigational product treatment / study treatment) and procedures specifying – when and how to withdraw subjects from the treatment, type and timing of the data to be collected from withdrawn subjects, whether and how subjects are to be replaced and the follow-up on the withdrawn subjects

(d) Statistical justification for the number of Subjects to be included in the Study

### *Handling of the Product(s)*

(a) Measures to be implemented to ensure the safe handling and storage of the pharmaceutical products.

(b) System to be followed for labelling of the product(s) (code numbering etc.)

(c) The label should necessarily contain the following information: the words - "For Clinical Studies only", the name or a code number of the study, name and contact numbers of the investigator, name of the institution, subject's identification code.

### *Assessment of Efficacy*

(a) Specifications of the parameters to be assessed to measure effects to be used

(b) Description of how effects are measured and recorded

(c) Time and periodicity of effect recording

(d) Description of special analyses and / tests to be carried out (pharmacokinetic, clinical, laboratory, radiological etc.)

### *Assessment of Safety*

(a) Specifications of safety parameters

(b) Methods and periodicity for assessing and recording safety parameters

(c) Procedures for eliciting reports of and for recording and reporting adverse drug reactions and / or adverse events and inter-current illnesses

(d) Type and duration of the follow-up of the subjects after adverse events

(e) Information on establishment of the study-code, where it will be kept and when, how and by whom it can be broken in the event of an emergency

*Statistics*

(a) Description of the statistical methods to be employed, including timing of any planned interim analysis

(b) Number of study subjects needed to achieve the study objective, and statistical considerations on which the proposed number of subjects is based

(c) Detailed break-up of the number of subjects planned to be enrolled at each study site (in case of multi-center studies)

(d) The level of statistical significance to be used

(e) Procedures for managing missing data, unused data and unauthentic data

(f) Procedures for reporting any deviations from the original statistical plan (any deviations from the original statistical plan should be stated and justified in protocol and / in the final report, as appropriate)

(g) Selection of the subjects to be included in the final analyses (e.g. all randomized subjects / all dosed subjects / all eligible subjects / evaluable subjects

### Data handling and management

A statement should be clearly made in the protocol that "The investigator(s) / institution(s) will permit study related monitoring, audits, ethics committee review and regulatory inspection(s) providing direct access to source data / documents".

A copy of the CRF should be included in the protocol. Besides, the following details should be given:

(a) Procedures for handling and processing records of effects and adverse events to the product(s) under study

(b) Procedures for the keeping of patient lists and patient records for each individual taking part in the study. Records should facilitate easy identification of the individual subjects.

## *Quality control and quality assurance*

(a) A meticulous and specified plan for the various steps and procedures for the purpose of controlling and monitoring the study most effectively

(b) Specifications and instructions for anticipated deviations from the protocol

(c) Allocation of duties and responsibilities within the research team and their co-ordination

(d) Instructions to staff including study description (the way the study is to be conducted and the procedures for drug usage and administration)

(e) Addresses and contact numbers etc. enabling any staff member to contact the research team at any hour

(f) Considerations of confidentiality problems, if any arise

(g) Quality control of methods and evaluation procedures

## *Finance and insurance*

(a) All financial aspects of conducting and reporting a study may be arranged and a budget is made out.

(b) Information should be available about the sources of economic support (e.g. foundations, private or public funds, sponsor / manufacturer). Likewise it should be stated how the expenditures should be distributed e.g. payment to subjects, refunding expenses of the subjects, payments for special tests, technical assistance, purchase of apparatus, possible fee to or reimbursement of the members of the research team, payment of the investigator / institution etc.)

(c) The financial arrangement between the sponsor, the individual researcher(s) / manufacturer involved, institution and the investigator(s) in case such information is not stated explicitly

(d) Study subjects should be satisfactorily insured against any injury caused by the study

(e) The liability of the involved parties (investigator, sponsor / manufacturer, institution(s) etc.) must be clearly agreed and stated before the start of the study

### Publication policy

A publication policy, if not addressed in a separate agreement, should be described in the protocol.

### Evaluation

(a) A specified account for how the response is to be evaluated

(b) Methods of computation and calculation of effects

(c) Description of how to deal with and the report of the subjects withdrawn from / dropped out of the study

### Supplementary and appendices

The following documents should be appended with the protocol:

(a) Information to the Study Subjects and the mode of providing it

(b) Instructions to staff

(c) Descriptions of special procedures

## Ethical and Safety Considerations

*The reader is requested to refer Ethical Issues in Clinical Trials for further details.*

### Ethical Principles

The following principles are to be followed:

(a) Principles of essentiality

(b) Principles of voluntariness, informed consent and community agreement

(c) Principles of non-exploitation

(d) Principles of privacy and confidentiality

(e) Principles of precaution and risk minimisation

(f) Principles of professional competence

(g) Principles of accountability and transparency

(h) Principles of the maximisation of the public interest and of distributive justice

(i) Principles of institutional arrangements

(j) Principles of public domain

(k)  Principles of totality of responsibility

(l)  Principles of compliance

## Ethics Committee

The sponsor and / or investigator should seek the opinion of an independent *Ethics Committee* regarding the suitability of the *Protocol*, methods and documents to be used in recruitment of *Subjects* and obtaining their *Informed Consent* including adequacy of the information being provided to the Subjects. The Ethics Committees are entrusted not only with the initial view of the proposed research protocols prior to initiation of the projects but also have a continuing responsibility of regular monitoring for the compliance of the Ethics of the approved programmes till the same are completed. Such an ongoing review is in accordance with the Declaration of Helsinki and all the international guidelines for biomedical research.

### *Basic Responsibilities*

The basic responsibility of an IEC is to ensure a competent review of all ethical aspects of the project proposals received and execute the same free from any bias and influence that could affect their objectivity.

The IECs should specify in writing the authority under which the Committee is established, membership requirements, the terms of reference, the conditions of appointment, the offices and the quorum requirements. The responsibilities of an IEC can be defined as follows:

(a)  To protect the dignity, rights and well being of the potential research participants.

(b)  To ensure that universal ethical values and international scientific standards are expressed in terms of local community values and customs.

(c)  To assist in the development and the education of a research community responsive to local health care requirements.

### *Special Considerations*

In addition to the usual requirements of biomedical research as a whole irrespective of the speciality of research, there are certain specific concerns pertaining to specialised areas of research which require additional safe guards / protection and specific considerations for the IEC. Examples of such instances are research involving children, pregnant and lactating women, vulnerable subjects and those with diminished autonomy besides issues pertaining to commercialisation of research and international collaboration. The observations and suggestions of IEC should be given in writing in unambiguous terms in such instances.

## Informed Consent Process

### *Informed Consent of Subject*

Prior to the beginning of the Study the Investigator(s) should obtain the Ethics Committee's approval for the written informed consent form and all information being provided to the subjects and / or their legal representatives or guardians as well as an impartial witness.

None of the oral and written information concerning the Study, including the written informed consent form, should contain any language that causes the subject(s) or their legal representatives or guardians to waive or to appear to waive their legal rights, or that releases or appears to release the Investigator, the Institution, the Sponsor or their representatives from their liabilities for any negligence.

The information should be given to the subjects and / or their legal representatives or guardians in a language and at a level of complexity that is understandable to the subject(s) in both written and oral form, whenever possible.

Subjects, their legal representatives or guardians should be given ample opportunity and time to enquire about the details of the study and all questions answered to their satisfaction.

The Investigator(s), sponsor or staff of the institution should not coerce or unduly influence a potential subject to participate or to continue to participate in the study. Careful consideration should be given to ensuring the freedom of consent obtained from members of a group with a hierarchical structure such as medical, pharmacy and nursing students, subordinate hospital and laboratory personnel, employees of the pharmaceutical industry, and members of the armed forces. Persons with incurable diseases, in nursing homes, in detention, unemployed or impoverished, in emergency rooms, homeless persons, nomads, refugees and any ethnic or racial minority groups should be considered as vulnerable population whose mode of consent should be carefully considered and approved by the Ethics Committee.

Prior to the subject's participation in the study the written Informed Consent form should be signed and personally dated by

1. (i) The subject *or* (ii) if the subject is incapable of giving an Informed Consent for example children, unconscious or suffering from severe mental illness or disability, by the subject's legal

representative or guardian *or* (iii) if the subject and his legal representative or guardian is unable to read / write;

2. An impartial witness who should be present during the entire informed consent discussion;

3. The Investigator.

By signing the consent form the witness attests that the information in the consent form and any other written information was accurately explained to, and apparently understood by, the Subject or the Subject's legal representative or the guardian, and that informed consent was freely given by the subject or the subject's legal representative or the guardian.

The subject's legal representative or guardian (if the subject is incapable of giving an Informed Consent for example children, unconscious or suffering from severe mental illness or disability), the inclusion of such patients in the study may be acceptable if the ethics committee is in principle, in agreement, and if the investigator thinks that the participation will promote the welfare and interest of the subject. The agreement of a legal representative or the guardian that participation will promote the welfare and interest of the subject should also be recorded with dated signature. If, however, neither the signed Informed Consent nor the witnessed signed verbal consent are possible – this fact must be documented stating reasons by the Investigator and also brought to the knowledge of Ethics Committee without any delay.

### *Essential information for prospective research on subjects*

Before requesting an individual's consent to participate in research, the investigator must provide the individual with the following information in the language he or she is able to understand, which should not only be scientifically accurate but should also be sensitive to their social and cultural context:

(i) The aims and methods of the research;

(ii) The expected duration of the subject participation;

(iii) The benefits that might reasonably be expected as an outcome of research to the subject or to others;

(iv) Any alternative procedures or courses of treatment that might be as advantageous to the subject as the procedure or treatment to which she/he is being subjected;

(v) Any foreseeable risk or discomfort to the subject resulting from participation in the study;

(vi) Right to prevent use of his/her biological sample (DNA, cell-line, etc.) at any time during the conduct of the research;

(vii) The extent to which confidentiality of records could be able to safeguard, confidentiality and the anticipated consequences of breach of confidentiality;

(viii) Free treatment for research related injury by the investigator / institution;

(ix) Compensation of subjects for disability or death resulting from such injury;

(x) Freedom of individual / family to participate and to withdraw from research any time without penalty or loss of benefits which the subject would otherwise be entitled to;

(xi) The identity of the research teams and contact persons with address and phone numbers;

(xii) Foreseeable extent of information on possible current and future uses of the biological material and of the data to be generated from the research and if the material is likely to be used for secondary purposes or would be shared with others, clear mention of the same;

(xiii) Risk of discovery of biologically sensitive information;

(xiv) Publication, if any, including photographs and pedigree charts.

The quality of the consent of certain social groups requires careful consideration as their agreement to volunteer may be unduly influenced by the Investigator.

## *Informed Consent in Non-Therapeutic Study*

In case of a Non-Therapeutic Study the consent must always be given by the subject. Non-Therapeutic Studies may be conducted in subjects with consent of a legal representative or guardian provided all of the following conditions are fulfilled:

1. The objective of the Study can not be met by means of a trial in Subject(s) who can personally give the informed consent

2. The foreseeable risks to the Subject(s) are low

3. Ethics Committee's written approval is expressly sought on the inclusion of such Subject(s)

### Essential Information on Confidentiality for Prospective Research Subjects Safe Guarding Confidentiality

The investigator must safeguard the confidentiality of research data, which might lead to the identification of the individual subjects. Data of individual subjects can be disclosed only in a court of law under the orders of the presiding judge or in some cases may be required to communicate to drug registration authority or to health authority. Therefore, the limitations in maintaining the confidentiality of data should be anticipated and assessed.

**Compensation for Participation**

Subjects may be paid for the inconvenience and time present, and should be reimbursed for expenses incurred, in connection with their participation in research. They may also receive free medical services. However, payments should not be so large or the medical services so extensive as to induce prospective subjects to consent to participate in research against their better judgement (inducement). All payments, reimbursement and medical services to be provided to the research subjects should be approved by the IEC. Care should be taken:

(i)   when a guardian is asked to give consent on behalf of an incompetent person, no remuneration should be offered except a refund of out of pocket expenses;

(ii)  when a subject is withdrawn from research for medical reasons related to the study the subject should get the benefit for the full participation;

(iii) when a subject withdraws for any other reasons he/she should be paid in proportion to the amount of participation.

Academic institutions conducting research in alliance with industries / commercial companies require a strong review to probe possible conflicts of interest between scientific responsibilities of researchers and business interests (e.g. ownership or part-ownership of a company developing a new product). In cases where the review board/committee determines that a conflict of interest may damage the scientific integrity of a project or cause harm to research participants, the board should advise accordingly. Institutions need self-regulatory processes to monitor, prevent and resolve such conflicts of interest. Prospective participants in research should also be informed of the sponsorship of research, so that they can be aware of the potential for conflicts of interest and commercial aspects of the research. Undue inducement through compensation for individual participants, families and populations should be prohibited. This prohibition, however, does not include agreements with individuals, families, groups, communities or populations that foresee technology transfer, local training, joint ventures, provision of health care reimbursement, costs of travel and loss of wages and the possible use of a percentage of any royalties for humanitarian purposes.

### Selection of Special Groups as Research Subject

#### *Pregnant or nursing women*

Pregnant or nursing women should in no circumstances be the subject of any research unless the research carries no more than minimal risk to the fetus or nursing infant and the object of the research is to obtain new knowledge about the foetus, pregnancy and lactation. As a general rule, pregnant or nursing women should not be subjects of any clinical trial except such trials as are designed to protect or advance the health of pregnant or nursing women or foetuses or nursing infants, and for which women who are not pregnant or nursing would not be suitable subjects.

(a) The justification of participation of these women in clinical trials would be that they should not be deprived arbitrarily of the opportunity to benefit from investigations, drugs, vaccines or other agents that promise therapeutic or preventive benefits. Example of such trials are, to test the efficacy and safety of a drug for reducing perinatal transmission of HIV infection from mother to child, trials for detecting fetal abnormalities and for conditions associated with or aggravated by pregnancy etc. Women should not be encouraged to discontinue nursing for the sake of participation in research and in case she decides to do so, harm of cessation of breast feeding to the nursing child should be properly assessed except in those studies where breast feeding is harmful to the infant.

(b) Research related to termination of pregnancy: Pregnant women who desire to undergo Medical Termination of Pregnancy (MTP) could be made subjects for such research as per The Medical Termination of Pregnancy Act, GOI, 1971.

(c) Research related to pre-natal diagnostic techniques: In pregnant women such research should be limited to detect the foetal abnormalities or genetic disorders as per the Prenatal Diagnostic Techniques (Regulation and Prevention of Misuse) Act, GOI, 1994 and not for sex determination of the foetus.

#### *Children*

Before undertaking trial in children the investigator must ensure that -

(a) children will not be involved in research that could be carried out equally well with adults;

(b) the purpose of the research is to obtain knowledge relevant to health needs of children. For clinical evaluation of a new drug the study in children should always be carried out after the phase III clinical trials in adults. It can be studied earlier only if the drug has a therapeutic value in a primary disease of the children;

(c) a parent or legal guardian of each child has given proxy consent;

(d) the assent of the child should be obtained to the extent of the child's capabilities such as in the case of mature minors, adolescents etc;

(e) research should be conducted in settings where the child and parent can obtain adequate medical and psychological support;

(f) interventions intended to provide direct diagnostic, therapeutic or preventive benefit for the individual child subject must be justified in relation to anticipated risks involved in the study and anticipated benefits to society;

(g) the child's refusal to participate in research must always be respected unless there is no medically acceptable alternative to the therapy provided/tested, provided the consent has been obtained from parents/guardian;

(h) interventions that are intended to provide therapeutic benefit are likely to be at least as advantageous to the individual child subject as any available alternative interventions;

(i) the risk presented by interventions not intended to benefit the individual child subject is low when compared to the importance of the knowledge that is to be gained.

### *Vulnerable groups*

Effort may be made to ensure that individuals or communities invited for research be selected in such a way that the burdens and benefits of the research are equally distributed.

(a) research on genetics should not lead to racial inequalities,

(b) persons who are economically or socially disadvantaged should not be used to benefit those who are better off than them,

(c) rights and welfare of mentally challenged and mentally differently able persons who are incapable of giving informed consent or those with behavioural disorders must be protected,

(d) Adequate justification is required for the involvement of subjects such as prisoners, students, subordinates, employees, and service personnel etc. who have reduced autonomy as research subjects.

## Compensation for Accidental Injury

Research subjects who suffer physical injury as a result of their participation in the Clinical Trial are entitled to financial or other assistance to compensate them equitably for any temporary or permanent impairment or disability subject to confirmation from IEC. In case of death; their dependents are entitled to material compensation.

### *Obligation of the sponsor to pay*

The sponsor whether a pharmaceutical company, a government, or an institution, should agree, before the research begins, to provide compensation for any serious physical or mental injury for which subjects are entitled to compensation or agree to provide insurance coverage for an unforeseen injury whenever possible.

## Responsibilities

### Sponsor

### *Investigator and Institution Selection*

The Sponsor is responsible for selecting the Investigator(s) / Institutions taking into account the appropriateness and availability of the study site and facilities. The Sponsor must assure itself of the Investigator's qualifications and availability for the entire duration of the Study. If organisation of a co-ordinating committee and / or selection of co-ordinating investigators are to be utilised in multi-centric studies their organisation and / or selection are Sponsor's responsibilities.

Before entering an agreement with an Investigator(s) / Institution(s) to conduct a Study, the Sponsor should provide the Investigator(s) / Institution(s) with the Protocol and an up-to-date Investigator's Brochure. Sponsor should provide sufficient time to review the protocol and the information provided in the Investigator's Brochure.

### *Contract*

The Sponsor should enter into a formal and legal agreement / contract with the Investigator(s) / Institution(s) on the following terms:

(a) To conduct the Study in compliance with GCP, the applicable regulatory requirements and the protocol agreed to by the sponsor and given approval / favourable opinion by the Ethics Committee;

(b) To comply with the procedures for data recording, and reporting;

(c) To permit monitoring, auditing and inspection;

(d) To retain the study related essential documents until the sponsor informs the Investigator(s) / Institution(s) in writing that these documents are no longer needed.

The agreement should define the relationship between the investigator and the sponsor in matters such as financial support, fees, honorarium, and payments in kind etc.

## Standard Operating Procedure

The sponsor should establish detailed Standard Operating Procedures (SOP's). The sponsor and the Investigator(s) should sign a copy of the Protocol and the SOPs or an alternative document to confirm their agreement.

### Allocation of duties and responsibilities:

Prior to initiating a study the sponsor should define and allocate all study related duties and responsibilities to the respective identified person(s) / organisation(s).

### Study management, data handling and record keeping:

The Sponsor is responsible for securing agreement with all involved parties on the allocation of protocol related and other responsibilities like:

(a) Access to all study related sites, source data / documents and reports for the purpose of inspection, monitoring and auditing by the authorised parties and inspection by national and foreign regulatory authorities

(b) Data processing;

(c) Breaking of the Code;

(d) Statistical analysis;

(e) Preparation of the study report;

(f) Preparation and submission of materials to the Ethics Committee, Regulatory Authorities and any other review bodies;

(g) Reporting the ADRs, AEs to the Ethics Committee;

(h) Quality Assurance and Quality Control systems with written SOPs to ensure that the study is conducted and data are generated, documented (recorded), and reported – in compliance with the Protocol, GCP and the applicable regulatory requirement(s).

It shall be the responsibility of sponsor to make arrangements for safe and secure custody of all study related documents and material for a period of three years after the completion of the study or submission of the data to the regulatory authority(ies) whichever is later.

The sponsor may consider establishing an Independent Data Monitoring Committee (IDMC) to assess the progress of the Study. This includes the safety data and the critical efficacy endpoints at various intervals, and to recommend to the sponsor whether to continue, modify, or stop a study. The IDMC should have written operating procedures and should maintain written records of all its meetings.

### Compensation for Participation

Subjects may be paid compensation for participation in accordance with the guidelines discussed earlier.

### Confirmation of review by the Ethics Committee

The sponsor shall obtain from the Investigator(s) and / or the Institutions

(a) The particulars about the members of the Investigator's / Institution's Ethics Committee including their names, addresses, qualifications and experience;

(b) An undertaking that the Ethics Committee is organised and operates according to the GCP and the applicable laws and regulations;

(c) Documented approval / favourable opinion of the Ethics Committee before the initiation of the Study;

(d) A copy of the recommendations in case the Ethics Committee conditions its approval upon change(s) in any aspect of the Study such as modification(s) of the Protocol, written Informed Consent Form, any other written information *and / or* other procedures;

(e) Ethics Committee's documents relating to re-evaluations / re-approvals with favourable opinion, and of any withdrawals or suspensions of approval / favourable opinion.

### Information on Investigational Products

As a prerequisite to planning of a study, the Sponsor is responsible for providing the Investigator(s) with an Investigator's Brochure. The Brochure must contain the available chemical, pharmaceutical, toxicological, pharmacological and clinical data including the available data from previous and ongoing clinical studies regarding the Investigational Product and, where appropriate, the Comparator Product. This information should be accurate and adequate to justify the nature, scale and the duration of the Study. In addition, the Sponsor must bring any relevant new information arising during the period of Study to the attention of the Investigator(s) as well as the Ethics Committee.

***Supply, storage and handling of Pharmaceutical Products***

The Sponsor is responsible for supplying the Investigational Product's, including Comparator(s) and placebo if applicable. The Products should be manufactured in accordance with the principles of GMPs and they should be suitably packaged in a manner that will protect the product from deterioration and safeguard blinding procedures (if applicable) and should be affixed with appropriate investigational labelling.

The sponsor should determine the Investigational Product's acceptable storage conditions, reconstitution procedures and devices for product infusions if any, and communicate them in writing to all involved parties, besides stating them on the Product labels wherever possible.

In case any significant formulation changes are made in the Investigational Product during the course of the study, the results of any additional studies of the new formulation (e.g. stability, bioavailability, dissolution rate) should be provided to the involved parties to enable them to determine their effects on the pharmacokinetic profile of the product prior to the use in the study.

The sponsor should not supply an Investigator / Institution with the product until the Sponsor obtains all required documentation (e.g. approval / favourable opinion from Ethics Committee and Regulatory Authorities).

The sponsor should document procedures and lay down responsibilities for

(a) adequate and safe receipt, handling, storage, dispensing of the Product;

(b) retrieval of unused product from the subjects and;

(c) return of unused product to the sponsor (or its alternative disposal procedure).

Sponsor should maintain records for retrieval of product (e.g. retrieval after study completion, expired product retrieval etc.).

Sponsor should also maintain records of the quantities of Investigational Product with proper batch numbers. The sponsor should ensure that the investigator is able to establish a system within his / her Institution for proper management of the products as per the procedures.

The sponsor should maintain sufficient samples from each batch and keep the record of their analysis and characteristics for reference, so that if necessary an independent laboratory may be able to recheck the same.

### Safety Information

Sponsor is responsible for the ongoing safety evaluation of the product. The sponsor should promptly notify findings to all concerned persons that could adversely affect the safety of the subjects, impact the conduct of the study or alter the Ethics Committee's approval / favourable opinion to continue the study. The sponsor, together with investigator(s), should take appropriate measures necessary to safeguard the study subjects.

### Adverse Drug Reaction Reporting:

The sponsor should provide ADR / AE reporting forms to the investigator(s) / institution(s). The sponsor should expedite the reporting to all concerned authorities (including the Ethics Committee and the regulatory authorities) of all serious and/or unexpected adverse drug reactions.

### Study Reports

The sponsor should ensure the preparation and appropriate approval(s) of a comprehensive final clinical study report suitable for regulatory and / or marketing purposes, whether or not the study has been completed. All reports prepared should meet the standards of the GCP guidelines for format and content of Clinical Study Reports. The sponsor should also submit any safety updates and / or periodic reports as prescribed by the regulatory authorities.

### Monitoring

Although an extensively written guidance can assure appropriate conduct of the study, the sponsor should ensure that the studies are adequately monitored. The determination of the extent and the nature of monitoring should be based on considerations such as objective, purpose, design, complexity, blinding, size and endpoints of the study. The sponsor must appoint adequately trained monitors or CRO to supervise an ongoing study.

### Audit

Sponsor should perform an audit as a part of QA system. This audit should be conducted with the purpose of being independent and separate from routine monitoring or quality control functions. Audit should evaluate the study conduct and compliance with the protocol, SOPs,

GCPs and applicable regulatory requirements. For the purpose of carrying out the audit, the sponsor may appoint individuals qualified by training and experience to conduct audits. The auditors should be independent of the parties involved in the study and their qualifications should be documented.

The sponsor should ensure that the auditing is conducted in accordance with the sponsor's SOPs on what to audit, how to audit, the frequency of audit and the form & content of audit reports. Auditors should document their observations which should be archived by the sponsors and made available to the Regulatory Authorities when called for.

Sponsor should initiate prompt action in case it is discovered that any party involved has not entirely complied with the GCP, SOPs, Protocol and / or any applicable regulatory requirements. If monitoring / auditing identifies serious and / or persistent non-compliance, the sponsor should terminate the defaulting party's participation in the study and promptly notify to the regulatory authority.

### *Multi-centre Studies*

Since multi-centre studies are conducted simultaneously by several investigators at different institutions following the same protocol, the sponsor should make special administrative arrangements for their conduct. These administrative arrangements should provide adequate assurance that the study will be planned and conducted according to GCPs.

The various tasks that may need special consideration include responsibility for commencement and overall performance of the study, supervision of the data, monitoring of the ADRs / AEs and various other policy matters. The functions, responsibilities and mandate of any special committee(s) set up or person(s) should be described in the study protocol, along with the procedure for their nomination.

A co-ordinating committee may be set up or a co-ordinator appointed with responsibility for the control of practical performance and progress of the study and maintaining contact with the regulatory authorities and the ethics committee(s).

Ideally, the studies should begin and end simultaneously at all institutions.

The sponsor should make arrangements to facilitate the communication between investigators at various sites. All investigators and other specialists should be given the training to follow the same protocol and systems. The sponsor should obtain written acceptance of the protocol and its annexes from each of the investigator and institution involved.

The CRFs should be so designed as to record the required data at all multi-centre sites. For those investigators who are collecting additional data, supplemental CRFs should be provided to record the additional data.

Before initiation of multi-centre studies the sponsor should carefully define and document the following:

(a) Ethics committee(s), and the number of ethics committees to be consulted;

(b) Role and responsibilities of the co-ordinating investigators;

(c) Role and responsibilities of the CRO;

(d) Randomisation procedure;

(e) Standardisation and validation of methods of evaluation and analyses of laboratory and diagnostic data at various centres;

(f) Structure and function of a centralised data management set-up.

### *Premature Termination or Suspension of a Study*

In case the sponsor chooses to or is required to terminate prematurely or suspend the study, then the sponsor should notify the investigator(s), institution(s), the ethics committee and the regulatory authorities accordingly. The notification should document the reason(s) for the termination or suspension by the sponsor or by the investigator / institution.

### *Role of Foreign Sponsor*

If the sponsor is a foreign company, organisation or person(s); it shall appoint a local representative or CRO to fulfil the appropriate local responsibilities as governed by the national regulations. The sponsor may transfer any or all of the sponsor's study related duties and functions to a CRO but the ultimate responsibility for the quality and the integrity of the study data shall always reside with the sponsor. Any study related duty, function or responsibility transferred to and assumed by a local representative or a CRO should be specified in writing. Any study related duties, functions or responsibilities not specifically transferred to and assumed by a CRO or a local representative shall be deemed to have been retained by the sponsor. The sponsor should utilise the services of qualified individuals e.g. bio-statisticians, clinical pharmacologists, and physicians, as appropriate, throughout all stages of the study process, from designing the protocol and CRFs and planning the analysis to analysing and preparing interim and final clinical study reports.

## Monitor

The monitor is the principal communication link between the sponsor and the investigator and is appointed by the sponsor.

### *Qualifications*

The monitor should have adequate medical, pharmaceutical and / or scientific qualifications and clinical trial experience. Monitor should be fully aware of all the aspects of the product under investigation and the protocol (including its annexes and amendments).

### *Responsibility*

The main responsibility of the monitor is to oversee the progress of the study and to ensure that the study conduct and data handling comply with the protocol, GCPs and applicable ethical and regulatory requirements.

(a) The Monitor should verify that the investigator(s) have the adequate qualifications, expertise and the resources to carry out the study. Monitor should also confirm that the investigator(s) shall be available throughout the study period.

(b) Monitor should ascertain that the institutional facilities like laboratories, equipment, staff, storage space etc. are adequate for safe and proper conduct of the study and that they will remain available throughout the study.

(c) The Monitor should verify (and wherever necessary make provisions to ensure) that:

1. The investigational product(s) are sufficiently available throughout the study and is stored properly;

2. The investigational product(s) are supplied only to subjects who are eligible to receive it and at the specified dose(s) and time(s);

3. The subjects are provided with the necessary instructions on proper handling of the product(s);

4. The receipt, use, return and disposal of the product(s) at the site are controlled and documented as prescribed;

5. The investigator receives the current Investigator's Brochure and all supplies needed to conduct the study as per the protocol;

6. The investigator follows the protocol;

7. The investigator maintains the essential documents;

8. All parties involved are adequately informed about various aspects of the study and follow the GCP guidelines and the prescribed SOPs;

9. Verifying that each party is performing the specified function in accordance with the protocol and / or in accordance with the agreement between the sponsor and the party concerned;

10. Verifying that none of the parties delegate any assigned function to unauthorised individuals.

(d) The monitor should promptly inform the sponsor and the ethics committee in case of any unwarranted deviation from the protocol or any transgression of the principles embodied in GCP.

(e) The monitor should follow a pre-determined written set of SOPs. A written record should be kept of the monitor's visits, phone calls and correspondence with the investigators and any other involved parties.

(f) The monitor should assess the institution(s)' facilities prior to the study to ensure that the premises and facilities are adequate and that an adequate number of subjects is likely to be available during the study.

(g) The monitor should observe and report the subject recruitment rate to the sponsor.

(h) The monitor should visit the investigator before, during and after the study to make assessments of the protocol compliance and data handling in accordance with the predetermined SOPs.

(i) The monitor should ensure that all staff assisting the investigator in the study have been adequately informed about and will comply with the protocol, SOPs and other details of the study.

(j) The monitor should assist the investigator in reporting the data and results of the study to the sponsor, e.g. by providing guidance on correct procedures for CRF completion and by providing data verification.

(k) The monitor shall be responsible for ensuring that all CRFs are correctly filled out in accordance with original observations, are legible, complete, and dated. The monitor should specifically verify that

1. The data required by the protocol are reported accurately on the CRFs and are consistent with the source documents;

2. Any dose and / or therapy modifications are well documented for each of the study subjects;

3. Adverse events, concomitant medications and inter-current illnesses are promptly reported on the CRFs in accordance with the protocol and the SOPs;

4. Visits that the subjects fail to make, tests that are not conducted and examinations that are not performed are clearly reported as such on the CRFs;

5. All withdrawals and drop-outs of enrolled subjects from the study are reported and explained on the CRFs.

(*l*) Any deviations, errors or omissions should be promptly clarified with the investigator, corrected and explained on the CRF. Monitor should also take appropriate actions designed to prevent recurrence of detected deviations. Monitor should ensure that investigator certifies the accuracy of CRF by signing it at the places provided for the purpose. All procedures for ensuring accuracy of CRFs must be maintained throughout the course of the study.

(m) The monitor should submit a written report to the sponsor after each site visit and after all telephone calls, letters and other correspondence with the investigator. Monitor's report should include the date, name of site, names of the monitor and the individuals contacted, a summary of what the monitor reviewed, findings, deviations & deficiencies observed, and any actions taken / proposed to secure compliance. The review and follow-up of the monitoring report with the sponsor should be documented by the sponsor's designated representative.

(n) The monitor should confirm that the prescribed procedures for storage, handling, dispensing and return of investigational product are being followed and their compliance is being documented in a form as in the SOPs.

## Investigator

### *Qualifications*

The investigator should be qualified by education, training and experience to assume responsibility for the proper conduct of the study and should have qualifications prescribed by the Medical Council of India (MCI). The investigator should provide a copy of the curriculum vitae and / or other relevant documents requested by the sponsor, the ethics committee, the CRO or the regulatory authorities. He / she should clearly understand the time and other resource demands the study is likely to make and ensure they can be made available throughout the duration of the study. The investigator should also ensure that other studies do not divert essential subjects or facilities away from the study at hand.

The investigator should be thoroughly familiar with the safety, efficacy and appropriate use of the investigational product as described in the protocol, investigator's brochure and other information sources provided by the sponsor from time to time.

The investigator should be aware of and comply with GCPs, SOPs and the applicable regulatory requirements.

### Medical care of the study subjects

A qualified Medical Practitioner (or a Dentist, when appropriate) who is an Investigator or a Co-Investigator for the study should be responsible for all study related medical decisions. Investigator has to ensure that adequate medical care is provided to a subject for any adverse events including clinically significant laboratory values related to the study. Investigator should inform the subject whenever medical care is needed for inter-current illness(es) of which the investigator becomes aware. Investigator should also inform the subject's other attending physician(s) about the subject's participation in the study, if the subject has another attending physician(s) and the subject agrees to such other physician(s). Subsequent to the completion of the study or dropping out of the subject(s) the investigator should ensure that medical care and relevant follow-up procedures are maintained as needed by the medical condition of the subject and the study and the interventions made.

Although a subject is not obliged to give reason(s) for withdrawing prematurely from a study, the investigator should make a reasonable effort to ascertain the reason(s) while fully respecting the subject's rights.

### Monitoring and Auditing of Records

The investigator / institution shall allow monitoring and auditing of the records, procedures and facilities, by the sponsor, the ethics committee, CRO or their authorised representative(s) or by the appropriate regulatory authority. The investigator should maintain a list of appropriately qualified person(s) to whom the investigator has delegated study-related duties.

Investigator should ensure that all persons involved in the study are adequately informed about the protocol, SOPs, the investigational product(s) and their study related duties and functions.

### *Communication with Ethics Committee*

Before initiating a study, the investigator / institution must ensure that the proposed study has been reviewed and accepted in writing by the relevant ethics committee(s) for the protocol, written informed consent form, subject recruitment procedures (e.g. advertisements) and any written / verbal information to be provided to the subjects.

The investigator should promptly report the following to the ethics committee, the monitor and the sponsor:

1. Deviations from or changes of, the protocol to eliminate immediate hazards to the subjects;

2. Changes that increase the risk to subject(s) and / or affecting significantly the conduct of the study;

3. All adverse drug reactions and adverse events that are serious and / or unexpected;

4. New information that may adversely affect safety of the subjects or the conduct of the study; and

5. For reported deaths the investigator should supply relevant additional information e.g. autopsy reports and terminal medical reports.

### *Compliance with the protocol*

The investigator / institution must agree and sign the protocol and / or another legally acceptable document with the sponsor, mentioning the agreement with the protocol, and confirm in writing that he / she has read and understood the protocol, GCPs and SOPs and will work as stipulated in them.

The investigator may implement a deviation from, or change of protocol to eliminate any immediate hazard(s) to the study subjects without prior ethics committee approval / favourable opinion. The implemented deviation or change, the reasons for it and if appropriate the proposed protocol amendment(s) should be submitted by the investigator to the ethics committee (for review and approval / favourable opinion), to the sponsor (for agreement) and if required to the regulatory authority(ies).

The investigator or person designated by him/her should document and explain any deviation from the approved protocol. The investigator should follow the study randomisation procedure, if any, and should ensure that the randomisation code is broken only in accordance with the protocol. If the study is blinded, the Investigator should promptly document and explain to the sponsor in case of any premature un-blinding (e.g. accidental un-blinding, un-blinding due to serious adverse event) of the Investigational Product(s) is done.

### Investigational Product(s)

Investigator has the primary responsibility for investigational product's accountability at the study site(s). Investigator should maintain records of the product's delivery to the study site, the inventory at the site, the use by each subject, and the return to the sponsor or the alternative disposal of the unused product(s). These records should include dates, quantities, batch / serial numbers, expiry dates if applicable, and the unique code number assigned to the investigational product packs and study subjects. Investigator should maintain records that describe that the subjects were provided the dosage specified by the protocol and reconcile all investigational products received from the sponsor. Investigator should ensure that the product(s) are stored under specified conditions and are used only in accordance with the approved protocol.

The investigator should assign some or all of his / her duties for investigational product's accountability at the study site(s) to his subordinate who is under the supervision of the investigator / institution. The investigator or subordinate should explain the correct use of the product(s) to each subject and should check at intervals appropriate for the study that each subject is following the instructions properly. The person who carries out them should document such periodic checks.

### Selection and recruitment of study subjects

The investigator is responsible for ensuring the unbiased selection of an adequate number of suitable subjects according to the protocol. It may be necessary to secure the co-operation of other physicians in order to obtain a sufficient number of subjects. In order to assess the probability of an adequate recruitment rate for subjects for the study, it may be useful to determine prospectively or review retrospectively, the availability of the subjects. Investigator should check whether the subject(s) so identified could be included in the study according to the protocol. The investigator should keep a confidential list of names of all study Subjects allocated to each study. This list facilitates the investigator / institution to reveal identity of the subject(s) in case of need and also serve as a proof of Subject's existence. The investigator / institution shall also maintain a Subjects' screening log to document identification of Subjects who enter pre-study screening. A Subject's enrolment log shall also be maintained to document chronological enrolment of Subjects in a particular Study.

The Investigator is responsible for giving adequate information to subjects about the trial in accordance with the GCP. The nature of the investigational product and the stage of development and the complexity of the study should be considered in determining the nature and extent of the information that should be provided.

### *Obligations of investigators regarding informed consent*

The investigator has the duty to:

1. Communicate to prospective subjects all the information necessary for informed consent. There should not be any restriction on subject's right to ask any questions related to the study, as any restriction on this undermines the validity of informed consent.

2. Exclude the possibility of unjustified deception, undue influence and intimidation. Deception of the subject is not permissible However, sometimes information can be withheld till the completion of the study, if such information would jeopardize the validity of research.

3. Seek consent only after the prospective subject is adequately informed. Investigator should not give any unjustifiable reasons to influence subject's decision to participate in the study.

4. As a general rule obtain from each prospective subject obtain a signed form as an evidence of informed consent (written informed consent) preferably witnessed by a person not related to the trial, and in case of incompetence to do so, a legal guardian or other duly authorised representative.

5. Renew the informed consent of each subject, if there are material changes in the conditions or procedures of the research or new information becomes available during the ongoing trial.

6. Not use intimidation in any form which invalidates informed consent. The investigator must assure prospective subjects that their decision to participate or not will not affect the patient-clinician relationship or any other benefits to which they are entitled.

As a part of the information provided to the Subject, the Investigator should supply subjects with, and encourage them to carry with them, information about their participation in the trial and information about contact persons who can assist in an emergency situation.

### *Records/Reports*

The investigator should ensure the accuracy, completeness, legibility, and timeliness of the data reported to the sponsor in the CRFs and in all required reports. Data reported on the CRF, that are derived from source documents, should be consistent with the source documents or the discrepancies should be explained.

Any change or correction to the CRF should be dated, signed and explained (if necessary) and should not obscure the original entry (i.e. an audit trial should be maintained); this applies to both written and electronic changes and corrections.

Sponsor should provide guidelines to investigators and / or the investigator's designated representatives on making such corrections and should have written procedures to assure that the changes in CRFs are documented and endorsed by the investigator. The investigator should retain records of the changes and corrections.

### *Progress Reports*

The investigator should submit the written summaries of the study status at the periodicity specified in the protocol, to the person(s) / organisation(s) to whom the investigator is reporting. All reportings made by the investigator should identify the subjects by unique code numbers assigned to the study subjects rather than by the subjects' name(s), personal identification number(s) and / or addresses.

### *Termination and final report*

In case the investigator and sponsor agree to prematurely terminate or suspend the study for any reason, the investigator / institution should promptly inform the study Subjects, the Ethics Committee as well as the Regulatory Authorities. The investigators should also ensure appropriate therapy and follow-up for the subjects.

However, if the investigator or the sponsor or the ethics committee decide to terminate or suspend the study without prior agreement of all parties concerned then the party initiating the suspension / termination should promptly inform all the concerned parties about such suspension / termination and suspension along with a detailed written explanation for such termination / suspension.

The Investigator should maintain documents as specified in the essential documents' list and take measures to prevent accidental or premature destruction.

The study can be closed only when the investigator (or the monitor or CRO – if this responsibility has been delegated to them) has reviewed investigator / institution and sponsor files and confirm that all necessary documents are in the appropriate files.

The completion of the study should be informed by the investigator to the institution, the sponsor and the ethics committee. The investigator should sign and forward the data (CRFs, results and interpretations, analysis and reports) of the study from his / her centre to the sponsor and the ethics committee. Collaborative investigators and those responsible for the analyses (including statistical analyses) and the interpretation of the results must also sign the relevant portions of the study report. Investigator should submit his signed and dated final report to the institution, the ethics committee and the sponsor, verifying the responsibility for the validity of data.

In case of a multi-centre study, the signature of the co-ordinating investigator may suffice, if agreed in the protocol.

In case the investigator is the sponsor then he / she assumes the responsibilities of both the functionaries.

The investigator should familiarise himself / herself with the various other responsibilities assigned to him/her under the protocol and ensure that they are carried out as expected.

## Record Keeping and Data Handling

The basic concept of record-keeping and handling of data is to record, store, transfer, and where necessary convert efficiently and accurately the information collected on the trial subject(s) into data that can be used to compile the study report.

### *Documentation*

All steps involved in data management should be documented in order to allow step-by-step retrospective assessment of data quality and study performance for the purpose of audit. Following the SOPs facilitates documentation.

Documentation SOPs should include details of checklists and forms giving details of actions taken, dates and the individuals responsible etc.

### Corrections

All corrections in the CRFs or any other study related documents should be made in a way that does not obscure the original entry. The correct data should be inserted along with the reason for the correction if such a reason is not obvious. The corrections should carry the date and initials of the investigator or the authorised person.

### Electronic Data Processing

For electronic data processing only authorised person should be allowed to enter or modify the data in the computer and there should be a recorded trail of the changes and deletions made. A security system should be set-up to prevent unauthorised access to the data. If data is altered during processing the alteration must be documented and the system should be validated. The systems should be designed to permit data changes in such a way that the data changes are documented and there is no deletion of data once entered. A list of authorised persons who can make changes in the computer system should be maintained. Adequate backup of the data should be maintained.

### Validation of Electronic Data Processing Systems

If trial data are entered directly into the computer there must always be an adequate safeguard to ensure validation, including a signed and dated printout and backup records. Computerised systems – hardware as well as software - should be validated and a detailed description of their use be produced and kept up-to-date.

### Language

All written documents, information and other materials used in the study should be in a language that is clearly understood by all concerned (i.e. the Subjects, paramedical staff, Monitors etc.)

### Responsibilities of the Investigator

Investigator should ensure that the observations and findings are recorded correctly and completely in the CRFs and signed by the responsible person(s) designated in the Protocol.

Laboratory values with normal reference ranges should always be recorded on a CRF or enclosed with the CRF. Values outside the clinically accepted reference range or values that differ significantly from previous values must be evaluated and commented upon by the Investigator. Data other than that requested by the Protocol may appear on the CRF clearly marked as the additional findings and their significance described by the investigator. Units of measurement must always be stated and transformation of units must always be indicated and documented.

In the medical records of the patient(s) it should be clearly indicated that the individual is participating in a clinical trial.

### *Responsibilities of the Sponsor and the Monitor*

The sponsor must ensure that electronic data processing system conforms to the certain documented requirements for completeness, accuracy, reliability and consistent intended performance (i.e. validation). The sponsor must maintain SOPs for using these systems. The monitor should take adequate measures to ensure that no data is overlooked. If the computer system automatically assigns any missing values, the fact should be clearly documented.

Sponsor should safeguard the blinding, if any, particularly during data entry and processing. The sponsor should use an explicit subject identification code that allows identification of all the data reported for each subject. Ownership of the data and any transfer of the ownership of data should be documented and intimated to the concerned party(ies).

## Quality Assurance

The sponsor is responsible for the implementation of a system of Quality Assurance in order to ensure that the study is performed and the data is generated, recorded and reported in compliance with the Protocol, GCP and other applicable requirements. Documented Standard Operating Procedures are a prerequisite for quality assurance.

All observations and findings should be verifiable, for the credibility of the data and to assure that the conclusions presented are correctly derived from the raw data. Verification processes must, therefore, be specified and justified.

Statistically controlled sampling may be an acceptable method of data verification in each study. Quality control must be applied to each stage of data handling to ensure that all data are reliable and have processed correctly.

Sponsor's audits should be conducted by persons independent of those responsible for the study. Investigational sites, facilities, all data and documentation should be available for inspection and audit by the Sponsor's auditor as well as by the Regulatory Authority(ies). *The reader is advised to see the separate chapter on Quality Assurance.*

## Statistics

### *Role of a Biostatistician*

Involvement of an appropriately qualified and experienced statistician is necessary in the planning stage as well as throughout the study. The Biostatistician should make a statistical model to help the sponsor, CRO and / or the Investigator in writing the Protocol. The number of subjects to be included in the study is determined in relation to the statistical model on which the protocol is based.

### *Study Design*

The scientific integrity of a clinical study and the credibility of its report depend on the design of the study. In comparative studies the protocol should describe:

1. An "a priori" rationale for the target difference between treatments that the study is being designed to detect, and the power to detect that difference, taking into account clinical and scientific information and professional judgment on the clinical significance of statistical differences.

2. Measures taken to avoid bias, particularly methods of Randomisation.

### *Randomisation and Blinding*

The key idea of a clinical trial is to compare groups of patients who differ only with respect to their treatment. If the groups differ in some other way, then the comparison of treatment gets biased. Randomisation, as one of the fundamental principles of experimental design, deals with the possible bias at the treatment allocation. It ensures that the allocation of treatment to human subjects is independent of their characteristics. Another important benefit of randomisation is that statistical methods of analysis are based on what we expect to happen in random samples from populations with specified characteristics. The protocol must state the method used for randomisation.

The study should use the maximum degree of blindness that is possible. Study subjects, investigator or any other party concerned with the study may observe and respond by knowledge of which treatment was given. To avoid such bias it is often desired that the patient or any other person involved in the study does not know which treatment was given. Where a sealed code for each individual treatment has been assigned in a blinded randomized study, it should be kept both at the site of the investigation and with the sponsor.

The Protocol must state the conditions under which the code is allowed to be broken and by whom. The system of breaking the code should be such that it allows access to only one subject's treatment at a time. The coding system for the investigational product(s) should include a mechanism that permits rapid identification of the products in case of a medical emergency, but does not permit undetectable breaks of the blinding.

### *Statistical Analysis*

The type(s) of statistical analyses to be used must be clearly identified and should form basis of the statistical model for the study. Any subsequent deviation(s) should be described and justified in the final report. The need and extent of an interim analysis must be specified in the protocol. The results of the statistical analyses should be presented in a manner that is likely to facilitate the interpretation of their clinical importance, e.g. by estimates of the magnitude of the treatment effect / difference and confidence intervals rather than sole reliance on significance testing.

Missing, unused and spurious data should be accounted for during the statistical analyses. All such omissions must be documented to enable review.

## Special Concerns

### Clinical Trials of Vaccines

### *Phases of Vaccine Trials*

The guidelines to conduct the clinical trial on investigational vaccines are similar to those governing a clinical trial. The phases of these trials differ from drug trials as given below:

*Phase I:* This refers to the first introduction of a vaccine into a human population for determination of its safety and biological effects including immunogenicity. This phase includes study of dose and route of administration and should involve low risk subjects. For example, immunogenicity to hepatitis vaccine should not be determined in high-risk subjects.

*Phase II:* This refers to the initial trials examining effectiveness (immunogenicity) in a limited number of volunteers. Vaccines can be prophylactic and therapeutic in nature. While prophylactic vaccines are given to normal subjects, therapeutic or curative vaccines may be given to patients suffering from a particular disease.

*Phase III:* This focuses on assessments of safety and effectiveness in the prevention of disease, involving controlled study on a larger number of volunteers (in thousands) in multi-centres.

### *Guidelines*

- The sponsor and investigator should be aware of the approval process(es) involved in conducting clinical trials of vaccines. They should familiarize themselves with the guidelines provided by Drug Controller General (India), Department of Biotechnology (DBT) and Ministry of Environment and Genetic Engineering Approval Committee (GEAC) in the case of vaccines produced by recombinant DNA technology.

- Some vaccines that contain active or live-attenuated microorganisms can possibly possess a small risk of producing that particular infection. The subjects to be vaccinated should be informed of the same.

- The subjects in control groups or when subjected to ineffective vaccines run a risk of contracting the disease.

- The risks associated with vaccines produced by recombinant DNA techniques are not completely known. However, for all the recombinant vaccines/products, the guidelines issued by the Department of Biotechnology should be strictly followed.

- Trials should be conducted by investigator with the requisite experience and necessary infrastructure for the laboratory evaluation of seroconversion.

- Protocols for such trials should include appropriate criteria for selection of subjects, plan of frequency of administration of the test vaccine in comparison with the reference vaccine. It should accompany detailed validation of testing method to detect the antibody titre levels.

- It should specify methodology to be adopted for prevention of centrifuged serum for the purpose of testing.

- The investigator should be provided with Quality Control data of the experimental batch of the vaccine made for the purpose of clinical trials.

- The sponsor should provide the Independent Ethics Committee approval of the nodal body (ies) to carry out clinical trials with the vaccine.

- The generic version of new vaccines already introduced in the other markets after step up clinical trials including extensive Phase III trials should be compared with the reference vaccine with regard to seroconversion in a comparative manner in a significant sample size.

- Post Marketing Surveillance (PMS) should be required following seroconversion studies. PMS data should be generated in a significant sample size sensitive to detect side effects and address other safety issues.

- Protocols for testing of new vaccine should contain a section giving details of steps of manufacture, in-process quality control measures, storage conditions, stability data and a flow chart of various steps taken into consideration in manufacturing of the vaccine. It should also contain detailed method of quality control procedure with the relevant references.

## Clinical Trials of Contraceptives

All procedures for clinical trials are applicable. Subjects should be clearly informed about the alternative available.

In women where implant has been used as a contraceptive for trial, a proper follow up for removal of the implant should be done, whether the trial is over or the subject has withdrawn from the trial.

Children born due to failure of contraceptives under study should be followed up for any abnormalities, if the woman does not opt for medical termination of pregnancy.

## Clinical trials with surgical procedures/ medical devices

Of late, biomedical technology has made considerable progress in the conceptualisation and designing of bio-equipments. Several medical devices and critical care equipments have been developed and many more are in the various stages of development. However, only through good manufacturing practices (GMP) the end products can reach the stage of utilization by society. Most of these products are only evaluated by

Central Excise testing for taxation purposes, which discourages entrepreneurs to venture out to this area with quality products especially when they do not come under the strict purview of the existing regulatory bodies like ISI, BSI and Drug Controller General. This is evidenced by the very low number of patents or propriety medical equipments manufactured and produced in the country. As the capacity of the country in this area is improving day by day, the need for a regulatory mechanism/ authority is increasingly obvious. The concept of regulations governing investigations involving biomedical devices is therefore relatively new in India. At present, except for needles and syringes these are not covered by the Drugs and Cosmetics Act, 1940. The Chief Executive of the Society of Biomedical Technology (SBMT) set up under the Defence Research Development Organisation (DRDO) has drafted a proposal for the setting up of a regulatory, tentatively named as the Indian Medical Devices Regulatory Authority (IMDRA). Until the guidelines are formulated and implemented by this regulatory authority, clinical trials with biomedical devices should be approved on case to case basis by committees constituted for the specific purpose.

### *Definitions*

*Medical devices:* A medical device is defined as an inert diagnostic of therapeutic article that does not achieve any of its principal intended purposes through chemical action, within or on the body unlike the medicated devices which contain pharmacologically active substances which are treated as drugs. Such devices include diagnostic test kits, crutches, electrodes, pacemakers, arterial grafts, intra-ocular lenses, orthopaedic pins and other orthopaedic accessories.

Depending upon risks involved, the devices could be classified as follows:

(a) *Non critical devices:* An investigational device that does not present significant risk to the patients: e.g. Thermometer, B.P. apparatus.

(b) *Critical devices:* An investigational device that presents a potential risk to the health, safety, welfare of the subject: for example, pacemakers, implants, internal catheters.

All the general principles of clinical trials described for drugs should also be considered for trials of medical devices. As for the drugs, safety evaluation and pre-market efficacy of devices for 1-3 years with data on adverse reactions should be obtained before pre-market certification. The duration of the trial and extent of use may be decided in case to case basis by the appropriate authorities. However, the following important factors that are unique to medical devices should be taken into consideration while evaluating the related research projects.

## *Guidelines*

- Safety data of the medical device in animals should be obtained and likely risks posed by the device should be considered.

- A clinical trial of medical devices is different from drug trials, as former cannot be done in healthy volunteers. Hence phase I of drug trial is not necessary for trial on devices.

- Medical devices used within the body may have greater risk potential than those used on or outside the body, for example, orthopaedic pins Vs crutches.

- Medical device not used regularly have less risk potential than those used regularly, for example, contact lens Vs intraocular lenses.

- Safety procedures to introduce a medical device in the patient should also be followed, as the procedure itself may cause harm to the patient.

- Informed consent procedures should be followed as in drug trials. The patient information sheet should contain information on following procedures to be adopted if the patient decides to withdraw from the trial.

## Clinical trials for Diagnostic Agents - Use of Radioactive Materials and X- Rays

In human beings, for investigation and treatment, different radiations: X-rays, gamma rays and beta rays, radio opaque contrast agents and radioactive materials are used. The relative risks and benefits of research proposal utilizing radioactive materials or X-rays should be evaluated. Radiation limits for the use of such materials and X-Rays should be in accordance with the limits set forth by the regulatory authority (BARC) for such materials. (BARC-Bhabha Atomic Research Centre, Mumbai).

### *Guidelines*

Informed consent should be obtained before any diagnostic procedures.

- Information to be gained should be gathered using methods that do not expose subjects to more radiation than exposed normally.

- Research should be performed on patients undergoing the procedures for diagnostic or therapeutic purposes.

- Safety measures should be taken to protect research subjects and others who may be exposed to radiation.

- The protocol should make adequate provisions for detecting pregnancies to avoid risks of exposure to the embryo.

- Information to subject about possible genetic damage to offspring should be given.

- Non-radioactive diagnostic agents are considered as drugs and the same guidelines should be followed when using them.

- Ultrasound to be submitted wherever possible.

### Clinical trials of Herbal Remedies and Medicinal Plants

For the herbal remedies and medicinal plants that are to be clinically evaluated for use in the Allopathic System and which may later be used in allopathic hospitals, the procedures laid down by the office of the DCG (I) for allopathic drugs should be followed. This does not pertain to guidelines issued for clinical evaluation of Ayurveda, Siddha or Unani drugs by experts in those systems of medicine, which may be used later in their own hospitals and clinics. All the general principles of clinical trials described earlier pertain also to herbal remedies. However, when clinical trials of herbal drugs used in recognized Indian systems of Medicine and Homoeopathy are to be undertaken in Allopathic Hospitals, associations of physicians from the concerned system as co-investigators/ collaborators/ members of the expert group is desirable for designing and evaluating the Study.

### *Categories of Herbal Products*

The herbal products can belong to any of the three categories given below:

(a) A lot is known about the use of a plant or its extract in the ancient Ayurveda, Siddha or Unani literature or the plant may actually be regularly used by physicians of the traditional systems of medicine for a number of years. The substance is being clinically evaluated for same indication for which it is being used or as has been described in the texts.

(b) When an extract of a plant or a compound isolated from the plant has to be clinically evaluated for a therapeutic effect not originally described in the texts of traditional systems or, the method of preparation is different, it has to be treated as a new substance or new chemical entity (NCE) and the same type of acute, subacute and chronic toxicity data will have to be generated as required by the regulatory authority before it is cleared for clinical evaluation.

(c) An extract or a compound isolated from a plant which has never been in use before and has not ever been mentioned in ancient literature, should be treated as a new drug, and therefore, should undergo all regulatory requirements before being evaluated clinically.

### *Guidelines*

- It is important that plants and herbal remedies currently in use or mentioned in literature of recognized Traditional System of Medicine is prepared strictly in the same way as described in the literature while incorporating GMP norms for standardization. It may not be necessary to undertake phase I studies. However, it needs to be emphasized that since the substance to be tested is already in use in the Indian Systems of Medicine or has been described in their texts, the need for testing its toxicity in animals has been considerably reduced. Neither would any toxicity study be needed for phase II trial unless there are reports suggesting toxicity or when the herbal preparation is to be used for more than 3 months. It should be necessary to undertake 4-6 weeks toxicity study in 2 species of animals in the circumstances pointed out in the preceding sentence or when a larger multicentric phase III trial is subsequently planned based on results of phase II study.

- Clinical trials with herbal preparations should be carried out only after these have been standardized and markers identified to ensure that the substances being evaluated are always the same. The recommendations made earlier regarding informed consent, subject, inducements for participation, information to be provided to the subject, withdrawal from study and research involving children or persons with diminished autonomy, all apply to trials on plant drugs also. These trials are also to be approved by the appropriate scientific and ethical committees of the concerned Institutes. However, it is essential that such clinical trials be carried out only when a competent Ayurvedic, Siddha or Unani physician is a co-investigator. It would neither be ethically acceptable nor morally justifiable, if an allopathic physician, based on references in ancient literature of above-mentioned traditional systems of Medicine, carries out clinical evaluation of the plant without any concept or training in these systems of medicine. Hence, it is necessary to associate a specialist from these systems and the clinical evaluation should be carried out jointly.

- When a Folklore medicine / Ethno-medicine is ready for commercialisation after it has been scientifically found to be effective, then the legitimate rights/ share of the Tribe or Community from whom the knowledge was gathered should be taken care of appropriately while applying for the Intellectual Property Rights and / Patents for the product.

## Key Points to Remember

- Good Clinical Practice provides guidelines of ethical and scientific quality standards for the design, conduct, recording and reporting of clinical research. Compliance of GCP ensures the adherence to the ethical and legal requirements.

- Compliance with GCP helps to ensure that the data generated are valid and accurate. In addition, it ensures that the research participants are not exposed to undue risks.

- GCP is based on Helsinki declaration. Indian GCP guideline was released in 2001.

- GCP describes: components of a study protocol, basic principles of ethics and functioning of human ethics committee, and responsibilities of all stake holders: sponsor, investigator, monitor, ethics committee etc.

- There are 12 basic principles of human ethics: principles of essentiality; principles of voluntariness, informed consent and community agreement; principles of non-exploitation; principles of privacy and confidentiality; principles of precaution and risks minimization; principles of professional competence; principles of accountability and transparency, principles of maximization of the public interest and of distributive justice; principles of institutional arrangements; principles of public domain; principles of totality of responsibility; and principles of compliance.

- The responsibilities of IEC are to ensure: complete reviewing of project proposal received; protecting the dignity, rights and well-beings of potential research participants; universal ethical values and international scientific standards; the development and the education of a research community responsive to local healthcare requirements.

- The responsibilities of sponsor are: identification of investigators and investigation sites; signing contract with investigators and the sites; developing detailed standard operating procedures for all operations; allocation of duties and responsibilities to the persons or institutions participating in the trial; study management, data handling, and record keeping; compensation for participation; get ethics committees approval; developing information on investigational products; supply, storage and handling of pharmaceutical products; managing and reporting of safety data; monitoring and auditing the study; and preparing final study report.

- The main responsibility of the monitor is to oversee the progress of the study and to ensure the study is being carried out in compliance with the protocol, GCP, ethical and legal requirements. Monitors have the enormous responsibilities as they are the eyes of the sponsor.

- The investigator is responsible for all study related medical decisions and ensures adequate medical care to the enrolled participants. Other responsibilities include: allowing monitoring and auditing; communicating with ethics committee; ensuring compliance with protocol, GCP and SOPs; keeping records of investigational products; selecting and recruiting study subjects; obtaining informed consents; accuracy of data; submitting progress reports; and the final report.

- Trials for vaccines, contraceptives, surgical procedures/medical devices, diagnostic agents and herbal medicines differ in some extent from that of clinical trial of pharmaceutical products. The basic principles remain same but there are additional requirements.

# CHAPTER 7

# Quality Assurance in Clinical Research

> Quality is never an accident; it is always the result of intelligent effort.
>
> J. Ruskin

**After reading this chapter, you should be able to:**

- Understand the concept and necessity of quality assurance in clinical research
- Importance of SOPs and how to write them
- Understand the concept of GCLP and its salient points.

The benefits of careful management of quality data in clinical research are well recognized. Maintaining accuracy and quality throughout a clinical study is a continual and dynamic process. Basically, it is the sponsor's responsibility to implement and maintain quality assurance and quality control systems with written Standard Operating Procedures (SOPs) to ensure that the trials are conducted and the data generated, documented and reported in compliance with the protocol, Good Clinical Practice (GCP) and applicable regulatory requirements.

The quality plan must be in place which includes both operational quality control and quality assurance activities. Operational quality control system defines standard for each key operational stage of the study against which quality control needs to be conducted. The quality assurance audit plan sets forth guidelines and expectations for the study and states the purpose and scope of audit schedule. The quality assurance audit plan too spells out what internal process of the study will be audited, from initial study design, site and data management, statistical analysis, and assembly of the final clinical study report. It specifies the organizational structure of audit team members and auditor for each study stage, as well as standards against which the audit will be conducted in terms of monitoring the original intent of the protocol, case report form completion guidelines, SOPs and GCP.

Every clinical research unit (contract research organization, also called as CRO) should have an appropriate Quality Assurance (QA) system. The QA system and the person(s) responsible for QA should operate independently of those involved in the conduct or monitoring of the trial. The QA unit should be responsible for:

- Verifying all activities undertaken during the study;
- Ensuring that QA systems, including SOPs of the CRO, are followed, reviewed and updated;
- Checking all the study data for reliability and traceability;
- Planning and performing self-inspections (internal audits) at regular and defined intervals in accordance with SOP, and following up on any corrective action as required;
- Ensuring that the contract facilities, such as analytical laboratories, adhere to good practices for quality control laboratories. This would include auditing of such facilities, and following up on any corrective action as required;
- Verifying that the trial report accurately and completely reflects the data of the study.

The CRO should allow the sponsor to monitor the studies and to perform audits of the clinical and analytical study and the sites. An audit of a clinical trial aims an independent review of quality data generated by the trial. The purpose of the audit is 'prevention, detection, and correction of errors, deviations or violations' to ensure validity of data and the integrity of clinical study. The functions of the audit include:

- Determining whether the rights and safety of the subjects have been adequately protected;

- Determining the level of compliance with GCP and applicable regulation;
- Preparing the site for regulatory inspections;
- Providing an independent assessment of trial activities;
- Helping achieve standardization and consistency of the process.

Though there are several other aspects to be carefully considered ensuring quality data output from clinical research, SOPs and Good Clinical Laboratory Practice (GCLP) and Data Management are undoubtedly the most important parameters. In the present text these three aspects are briefly discussed.

## SOPs – a Tool to Implement GCP

Standard Operating Procedures (SOPs) are standard, elaborate, written instructions to achieve uniformity of performance in all the tasks related to a function (Clinical Trial). They define responsibilities, specify records to be established and maintained, and specify methods and procedures to be used in carrying out study related activities. SOPs coupled with close personal supervision of the trial's conduct by the investigator and carefully monitoring by the sponsor help to ensure that processes are consistently followed and activities are consistently documented. SOPs form the basis of GCP compliant clinical trial by allowing uniformity and standardization of tasks and by fulfilling the regulatory requirements. If SOPs are not followed correctly, the validity of data generated is doubtful. Every one involves in the trial like sponsor, investigator, ethics committee, regulator is required to follow SOPs pertaining to the individual's task.

Sponsor is required to prepare, follow and document SOPs on the conduct of trial related activities, process of data management, record keeping, and internal QA & QC processes.

The investigator is required to comply with sponsor's SOPs while conducting the clinical trial. The site is required to have its own SOPs in agreement with sponsor's SOPs for various activities related to study such as source data management, screening, enrolment, IC process, subject management while on study, AE and SAE reporting and handling, specimen collection and dispatch, IP management, CRF management, archiving etc. EC is required to prepare, follow and document its own SOPs on number selection process, duties of EC members, functioning and operation of EC including frequency of meetings, review process, method of communication or notification. The regulators (CDSCO/DCGI) should have the SOPs for keeping record of all trials and activities under taken by each stake holder. This would facilitate inspection and auditing.

In short SOPs are the tools to implement GCP to ensure that the data collected should ordinarily be reliable enough for regulatory decision making. It addresses the who, what, when, how and why of clinical research operations.

The SOPs should have the following attributes:

- Comprehensive, practical and customised: It should contain just relevant (not too much), practical and specific information required to perform function.

- Thorough: It must be thorough enough for easy understanding (not giving scope to assume or presume) and implementation.

- Dynamic: The SOPs are likely to change depending upon need and due to scientific or regulatory development. Hence they must have flexibility for changing.

- Robust: It should be strong enough to allow easy transfer to other personnel or laboratories. Each department of the organization should develop own SOPs depending on its function or activities.

The writing of SOP is not an easy process and is very time consuming, but pays big dividends when complete. Developing SOPs is very critical as this defines the activities of the organization. There are different types of SOPs each of which has its own merits and demerits:

- Simple Steps
- Hierarchical Steps
- Graphics
- Enhanced Graphics
- Flowcharts

The writing and management of SOPs involve the following steps:

1. **Mapping the SOP**: It is first necessary to study and understand the procedures for which the SOP is to be written. A previously developed SOP is often helpful. Process mapping involves laying out all steps involved and analyzing the process with a goal of making it more efficient and easier to follow. All the persons involved in doing a particular task should be involved in mapping it into a process chart.

   A simple flow chart describing what is done at each step including the critical "hows" must be written. This sketch helps in developing the actual SOP using the official template.

   The SOPs are required to be written for all aspects of Clinical Trial: protocol preparation, ethical approval, assessing and monitoring trial sites, safety data reporting, checking data integrity, clinical report writing, database preparation, validating computer systems etc..

   Though there are no fixed formats for writing SOPs, it is necessary that the procedures are presented in a format that will work for the institution and address the specific needs. The goal is to have easily understood procedure that the clinical research staff will clearly understand and utilize. The SOPs should have atleast the following templates:

   *Category*: Administrative/Study Conduct/Ethical Review etc.

   *Title*: Should be descriptive. It should give a clear indication of the activity which it describes.

   *SOP Number*: There should be numbering system for each organization.

   *Version*:

   *Total Pages*: Each page has to be numbered as X of Y.

   *Validity*: With effective date and review date.

   *Author*:

   *Reviewer*:

   *Approved by with date of approval*:

***Distribution***: No superseded or obsolete SOPs should be made available at user points. Each time a SOP is reviewed and amended, superseded versions of SOPs should be removed from all user points and replaced with updated version. The list of distribution is maintained.

***Objective***: This describes what is to be accomplished and/or achieved with this SOP.

***Responsibilities***: This describes the persons responsible to perform the activity or follow SOP. It is preferable to write the position (designation) rather than name of the person.

***Scope***: This describes the areas this procedure does and does not apply.

***Reference to other applicable SOPs***: This describes the SOPs which may provide additional information for this SOP.

***Appendices***: They are attachments.

***Flow Chart***: This summarises the steps.

***Procedure or Instruction***: This describes the step by step description with instruction for completing the task.

A major decision is necessary in defining the level of detail that should be incorporated in writing SOP. In general, the higher levels of details are required:

- When the task is infrequently performed.
- When the task is critical.
- If different people are involved.
- If low variation is allowed in performance.
- Training is not comprehensive or there is less time to practice the task.

2. **Use of Language and Writing the SOP:**

The SOPs must be written in a clear unambiguous language that can be easily understood by the users. The important tips for writing SOPs include:

- Use short and active sentences:  Do -------.
- Use simple words.

- Write instruction in right order to make the operator understand when to do the task.
- Make use of diagram for easy understanding wherever possible.
- Limit the quantum of information per page (Do not overload).
- Mention the references at the end.

3. **Checking of the Draft SOP:** The draft SOP is required to be checked for style and format, edition number, correctness and consistency for contents, compliance with policy, GCP and regulatory requirements.

4. **Approval of SOP:** After formal checking or review of the draft SOP (after correction), the SOP is to be approved for adoption. This authorization is usually done by the designated official who has good insight of the organization and the GCP.

5. **Distributing and Retrieving:** The designated official or staff in the organization should be identified who would be responsible for distribution of SOP. Records of distribution and retrieval of SOPs should be maintained to ensure that superseded SOPs are still not in use. A copy of original SOP is to be made and stamped as "Official Copy" in red ink. The official copies of SOPs are only controlled.

When the SOP is reviewed and amended, copies of superseded SOP should be retrieved from all those who hold a copy when the new version is distributed. The original SOP should be marked as "superseded" on each page and file in the "superseded file". The retrieved superseded SOPs should be destroyed.

6. **Training on SOP:** The training of individuals who would be using the SOP is an important step in effective implementation of SOP. This needs to be completed before the effective date of SOP. Normally the quality assurance staff are responsible for giving the training. The training should be documented and must be recorded in staff training record.

7. **Implementation and Maintenance:** The SOP is implemented on the date specified after distribution and training. The mechanism must be made available to ensure that only approved version is in

circulation. No individual is allowed to manipulate the SOP. When a mistake is found, it should be brought to the notice of the designated official and never to correct it individually. The detection of mistake is an indicator of need of updating SOP.

8. **Review of SOP:** A date should be assigned on which the SOP will be reviewed to determine whether any changes are required to keep it up to date. Each SOP should have a time limit for validity and should be reviewed before the end of the period of validity. The updated SOP should go through the same writing and revision process.

| List of SOPs required during Clinical Trial or Bioequivalence Study (not exhaustive) | |
|---|---|
| SOP for writing SOP | Payment to research subjects |
| Conduct of Study | Procedures for entry into and exit from clinical unit |
| Achieving and Retrieval of Documents related to study | Handling of subject check- in and check – out |
| QA of the study including auditing of clinical and bioanalytical part of the study and the study report | House keeping at clinical unit |
| Study files | Planning, preparation, evaluation and service of standardized meals for study subjects |
| Preparation and review of the protocol for the study | Distribution of meals to subjects |
| Amendment to the protocol for the study | Operation and maintenance of nurse calling system |
| Protocol deviations/violation recording and reporting | Administration of drugs to subjects |
| Sponsor/CRO quality assurance agreement in conducting the study | Cannulation of study subjects |
| Study approval process by ethics committee | Collection of blood samples from study subjects |
| Study report | System for number of bio-samples |
| Written informed consent | Recording of vital signs of subjects |
| Obtaining written informed consent for screening from study subjects | Operation and verification of fire alarm system |
| Allotment of identification number to study | Oxygen administration to subject |

| | |
|---|---|
| subjects | |
| Investigator's brochure | Emergency care of subjects during study |
| Case report form | Availability of ambulance during study |
| Preparation of case report form, review and completion | Centrifugation and separation of blood samples |
| Data collection and case report form completion | Storage of plasma/serum samples |
| Adverse/serious adverse reaction/event monitoring, recording and reporting | Segregation of bio-samples |
| Organization chart of the study | Transfer of plasma/serum samples to bioanalytical laboratory |
| Training of the personnel | Procedures for washing glassware |
| Responsibilities of the members of the research team | Recording temperature and relative humidity of rooms |
| Monitoring of the study by the sponsor | Introduction on of operation and maintenance procedures for all the equipments in the clinical unit |
| Conduct of pre-study meeting | Numbering the equipments and maintenance of logbook |
| Study start up | Control of access to pharmacy |
| Subject management | Pharmacy area requirements |
| SOP on mobilization of individuals for registration into volunteer bank | Investigational drug supply management |
| Eligibility criteria for registration and registration of individuals into volunteer bank | Study drug receipt, return and accountability documentation |
| Handling of subject withdrawal | Study of drug receipt and return procedure |
| Allotment of identification number to study subjects | Retention of samples of study drugs |
| Screening of enrolled subjects for the study | Disposal of achieved study drugs |
| Collection of urine samples of subjects for detection of drugs of abuse and transportation of samples to pathology laboratory | Disposal of biological materials |
| Custodian duties | Procedures for bioanalytical laboratory (SOP for different equipment, analytical methods, reagent preparation) |
| Data analysis from Analytical data | Out of specification situation in the laboratory |

| Statistics in the study | Acceptance criteria for analytical runs based on QC sample results |
|---|---|
| Site Master file management | Chromatographic acceptance criteria, chromatogram integration |
| Investigator selection | Sample re-assay |
| Regulatory submission | |
| Obtaining ethics committee approval (submission of document to receiving approval) | |

Source: Suitably modified from WHO Expert Committee on Specifications for Pharmaceutical Preparations, 40th Report, WHO, Geneva, 2006.

## Example of a SOP

**Category: Study Conduct**
**Title: Breaking Code**

**SOP No: GPM CT/1;**                                     **Version: August 2010**

**SOP Author: Dr. Guru Prasad Mohanta**

**Reviewed by: Dr. XYZ**

**Approved by: Dr. ZYX**                    **Date of Approval: 01 August 2010**

**Effective Date: 15 August 2010**              **Review Date: 14 August 2011**

**Number of Pages:02**

---

**Title**: Breaking Code

**Scope:** Applicable to Phase – I, II and III clinical trials which are blinded to investigators. The blind is to be broken on an individual basis due to a medical emergency including the occurrence of severe adverse event.

**Responsibilities:** The clinical trial monitor or clinical trial coordinator or product manager are responsible for breaking the code.

**Objective:** To define the circumstances under which individual subject randomization may be broken in the case of a medical emergency and how to document this event.

**Reference to other SOPs:**

1.  SOP No. ---: Responsibilities of clinical trial monitor.
2.  SOP No. --: Adverse Event Monitoring, Assessment and Reporting.
3.  SOP No. ---: Study randomization

**Procedure:**

1.  Ensure that the investigator knows that the code break will be performed only in the event of medical emergency, when the physician in charge of the subject feels that the subject cannot be treated adequately unless the identity of the investigation product is known or the information is essential for further management of the other subjects.

2.  Emphasize the investigator to make every effort to contact the sponsor/clinical trial monitor prior to breaking the code. If this is not possible, and the situation is an emergency, the investigator may break the code and contact the trial monitor as soon as possible thereafter.

**Category: Study Conduct**
**Title: Breaking Code**

**SOP No: GPM CT/1;**                    **Version: August 2010**
**SOP Author: Dr. Guru Prasad Mohanta**
**Reviewed by: Dr. XYZ**
**Approved by: Dr. ZYX**         **Date of Approval: 01 August 2010**
**Effective Date: 15 August 2010**     **Review Date: 14 August 2011**
**Number of Pages:02**

Following a request either from investigator or physician, the individual code for the subject should be broken and the investigator or physician be informed. Document the following:

- Protocol number
- Study number
- Subject number
- Date of code break
- Identification and signature of the person breaking the code
- Identification of the person requesting the code break
- Reason (s) for breaking code
- Investigator's signature

❖ Record all the information on an emergency code break form and on the case report form.

❖ If the randomization code was not declared in the investigator's initial serious adverse experience report, update the serious adverse experience worksheet once the blind is broken for the study.

❖ Ensure that the clinical data management personnel are informed.

❖ Ensure that all documentation relating to the code break is included in the study file.

**Distribution:**                    **Received by:**

## Good Clinical Laboratory Practice (GCLP)

The laboratory investigations are integral part and used to support clinical research. The investigation results, therefore, should be reliable, accurate and reproducible. The generation of such quality results involves a stepwise process of meticulous planning, perfect execution and thorough checking of the results by the whole research team. The GCLP guideline outlines the principles and procedures to be followed by medical or clinical laboratories involved in the clinical research so as to ensure generation of quality data and facilitate the acceptance of clinical data by regulatory authorities from around the world. GCLP applies those principles established under Good Laboratory Practices (GLP) for data generation and is used in regulatory submissions relevant to the analysis of samples from clinical trial. GCLP should be followed by all laboratories involve in the analysis of biological samples ranging from routine safety monitoring of volunteers to bioavailability research.

*GLP*: is a managerial concept covering the organizational process and the conditions under which the laboratory studies are planned, performed, monitored, recorded and reported, aiming to promote quality and validity of test data.

*GCLP*: applies the GLP principles to the analysis of samples from a clinical trial to ensure generation of reliable and credible results acceptable to regulatory authorities.

The salient points of GCLP include (It is not the full guideline):

### A. Organization and Personnel:

1. **Responsibilities of Trial Facility Management**: The trial facility management should ensure or maintain -

   - Availability of  qualified personnel, appropriate facilities, equipment, and materials;
   - Record of the qualifications, training, experience and job description for each individual working within the trial facility;
   - Clear understanding of the job by the persons employed;
   - Availability of health and safety precautions within the trial facility, based on national and / or international regulations;
   - Development and adoption of appropriate standard operating procedure (SOP) and archival of previous SOPs;
   - Working of quality audit programme with designated personnel;
   - Operation of quality control programme;

- Existence of analytical plan for the proposed analysis and mechanisms to its amendment;
- Maintenance of copies of trial protocol and analytical plans;
- Availability of sufficient number of personnels for timely and proper conduct of the work;
- Appointment of Analytical Project Manager with appropriate qualification, training and experience, before the initiation of trial;
- Availability of the identified personnel for the management of the archives used for the retention of trial and facility records.

2. **Responsibilities of Analytical Project Manager:**
   - Overall conduct of analyses performed by the trial facility and its reporting;
   - Agreeing to analytical plan;
   - Ensuring the adoption of analytical plan; authorizing the change in the plan if required;
   - Ensuring the documentation of all results of analyses;
   - Signing with date, indicating acceptance of responsibility for the validity of the results and confirming compliance with GCLP; Ensuring that the data are released only under dated signature;
   - Ensuring, archiving and retaining all analytical results including raw data and supporting documents on completion of the analyses.

3. **Responsibilities of Trial Staff:**
   - They must be aware of these guidelines and follow the instructions given in the trial protocol, analytical plans and SOPs. They are responsible for the quality of data.

**B. Facilities:**

1. **Trial Facility should have:**
   - Suitable size, construction and location to meet the requirements of the trial and minimize any disturbances that might interfere with the validity of the trial; (Appropriate size area should be available for performing the work and provide security to assure integrity of trial samples at all times).

- Suitable facilities for the preparation of trial supplies, to ensure accuracy of preparations;

- Appropriate storage areas required for samples and supplies. Storage area should be separate to prevent contamination or mix up of trial samples or materials.

### 2. Archive Facility:

- Appropriate space should be made available for safe and secure archive storage and retrieval of data, reports, samples and specimens. Alternatively a third party contract can be given for this purpose.

### 3. Waste Disposal:

- The handling and disposal of wastes generated during the trial should be carried out in a manner that is consistent with national guideline [Biomedical Waste (management and handling) rules 1998 as amended in 2000.

## C. Equipment, Material and Reagents:

### 1. Equipment:

- The equipment must be of appropriate design and capacity and suitably located.

- The equipment used should be periodically inspected, cleaned, maintained and calibrated. The record of such activities should be maintained and retained.

- Suitably qualified and trained persons should be made available for operating the equipment.

### 2. Material:

- The materials should be of appropriate quality.

### 3. Reagents:

- Reagents should have suitable label indicating the identity, concentration, specific storage requirements including the date of preparation and date of expiry.

**D. Standard Operating Procedures (SOPs):**

The bio-analytical laboratory should have SOPs for all its activities. The following SOPs are essential:

1. **Trial Supplies:** Supply, preparation, labeling, handling, shipment and storage.

2. **Equipment:** Operation, maintenance, cleaning, calibration.

3. **Record Keeping, Reporting, Storage, and Retrieval:** Coding of trials, data collection, preparation of reports, indexing systems, handling of data, use of computer data systems and operation of archieves.

4. **Trial Materials:** Storage, retrieval and custody of samples.

5. Preparation of Trial Packs.

6. Procedure for receipt, transfer, sampling, storage, identification and care of trial materials and samples.

7. Procedures for analysis of trial samples.

8. **Quality Control Procedures:** to ensure the quality and accuracy of results.

9. **Quality Audit Procedures:** Operation of quality audit personnel in performing and reporting trial audits, inspections and analytical report reviews.

**The two important tools required for maintaining laboratory quality:**

1. Internal Quality Control – for detection and minimization of immediate errors

2. External Quality Assessment – for monitoring long term precision and accuracy of results.

## Data Management

The primary objective of clinical data management is to ensure timely delivery of high quality data which are necessary to satisfy or comply: GCP requirements, Statistical Analysis and Reporting (Regulatory) Requirements. The data management begins when the protocol is written and the data capture tool is designed, and continues through the study drug being approved for marketing and beyond into PMS.

The sponsor may consider establishing an Independent Data Monitoring Committee to assess the progress of a clinical trial, including the safety data and critical efficacy end points at intervals, and to recommend to the sponsor whether to continue, modify, or stop a trial.

The Data Monitoring Committee should have written operating procedures and maintain written records of all its meetings. While the data management in clinical trials itself is a big business, the sponsor often outsources this activity to information technology experts or companies. The thorough discussion of this aspect of clinical trials is beyond the scope of this text. The readers are encouraged to refer various texts available.

The collection of data and transfer of data from investigator to sponsor can take place through a various media, including paper case records form, remote site monitoring systems, medical computer systems and electronic transfer. Whatever data capture instrument is used, the form and the content of the information collected should be in full accordance with the protocol and should be established in advance of the conduct of clinical trials. It should focus on data necessary to implement the planned analysis, including the context information necessary to confirm protocol compliance or identify important protocol deviations. 'Missing values' should be distinguishable from the 'value zero' or 'characteristic absent'. The missing data represent a potential source of bias in a clinical trial. Hence, every effort should be undertaken to fulfill all the requirements of the protocol concerning the collection and management of data. In reality, however, there will almost always be some missing data. There should be predefined methods included in the protocol to deal with the missing data. The process of data capture through to data base finalization should be carried out in accordance with the GCP.

When using electronic trial data handling and/ or remote electronic trial data system, the sponsor should:

- Ensure and document that the electronic data processing system(s) confirms to the sponsor's established requirements for completeness, accuracy, reliability, and are consistent with intended performance.

- Maintain SOPs for using this system.

- Ensure that the systems are designed to permit data changes are documented and that there is a way that the data changes are documented and there is no deletion of entered data.

- Maintain a security system that prevents unauthorized access to the data.

- Maintain a list of the individuals who are authorized to make data changes.
- Maintain adequate back up of the data.
- Safeguard the blinding during data entry and processing.

The decision to transform key variables prior to analysis is best made during the design of the trial on the basis of similar data from earlier clinical trials. In such situation, the provision should be available to compare the original data and observations with the processed data.

In addition, sponsor has the following responsibility towards data management:

- Using unambiguous subject identification code that allows identification of all the data reported, for each subject.
- Retaining all documents pertaining to clinical trials and other records in conformance with regulatory requirements.
- Retaining all documents for at least two years after formal discontinuation of a trial or in conformance with regulatory requirements.
- Notifying all investigators, institutions, and regulatory authorities, if the trial is discontinued.
- Reporting the transfer of ownership of data to the appropriate authority, in case ownership transfer is made.
- Retaining the essential documents of the trials to such a period as required after marketing approval.
- Informing the investigator(s) and the institution(s) in writing the need for record retention and when the trial related records are no longer needed.

The credibility of numerical results of the data interpretation (results) depends on the quality and validity of the methods and software used for data management (data entry, storage, verification, correction, and retrieval) and also processing the data statistically. The computer software used for data management and statistical analysis should be reliable and hence is necessary to validate prior to use.

The readers are advised to see the chapter on data management for more details.

**NABH-Accreditation Standards**: In 2014, the National Accreditation Board for Hospitals and Healthcare Providers, a constituent body of Quality Council of India, has issued draft accreditation standards for clinical trial site, ethics committee and investigators. Criteria or Parameters for assessment:

- **Ethics Committee:** Composition, procedures for new induction and resignation of members; Frequency of ethics committee meetings; Receipt, review and decision making of proposals; Review of protocol amendments; Procedure for deliberations and maintaining minutes; Periodic review and oversight; Procedure to be followed for vulnerable population; Review of Informed consent document (subject information sheet and informed consent form) and informed consent process; Reporting, analysis of SAEs and making opinion on compensation; Handling issues related to non-compliances, protocol violation, complaints by the participants and other stakeholders; Declaration of conflict of interest and confidentiality agreement; Financial declaration of payments received and disbursed; Training for committee members; Communication with different stakeholders; Control and archiving of records; and SOP on SOP.

- **Investigator:** Investigator roles and responsibilities; Investigator education, qualification and experience; adherence to site SOPs and study protocol for all essential trial activities; procedures on informed consent, safety reporting and management, delegation of responsibilities and training, investigational product, protocol compliance and protocol deviations, clinical trial documentation, records retention and archival and destruction.

- **Clinical Trial Site:** Subject protection policy (including transparent mechanism of enrollment and continuity of care of subjects in clinical trials); Informed consent, including procedures for audio-visual recording of consent; Medical management of adverse events; Adverse events and serious adverse events reporting (including emergency care) and compensation for trial injury; Roles and responsibilities of study team; Site research team training; Research pharmacy (investigational product management); Protocol compliance and protocol deviations; Documentation policy; Storage and retention of trial related documents; Conflict of interest disclosure policy; Resources (access to adequate laboratory facilities, adequate space and required medical and paramedical personnels, adequate arrangement for volunteers, subjects for isolation, recreation, food, as applicable); Equipment calibration and maintenance; Quality management plan (including quality control measures); and Oversight by Ethics Committee.

# Key Points to Remember

- Maintaining accuracy and quality throughout the clinical study is a continual and dynamic process. It is the sponsor's primary responsibility to implement and maintain quality assurance and quality control system with written Standard Operating Procedure (SOP).

- Every clinical research unit should have a quality assurance unit which is responsible for ensuring adherence to SOPs and quality assurance protocol.

- Monitoring and auditing of clinical trials, analytical study and clinical trial sites should be conducted to ensure compliance with study protocol and GCP.

- SOPs are important tools to implement GCP. They define the responsibilities, specify records and their maintenance, and specify methods and procedures to be followed in carrying out clinical trials. All stake holders should have their own SOP for each activity.

- The qualities of SOPs are: comprehensive; practical, customized; thorough; dynamic; and robust.

- Development of SOPs involve the following steps: mapping the SOP; use of language and writing the SOP; checking the draft SOP; approval of SOP; distributing and retrieving; training on SOP; implementation and maintenance; and reviewing of SOP.

- Good Clinical Laboratory Practice (GCLP) is to be followed for all laboratory investigations associated with clinical research. The GCLP guideline outlines the principles and procedures to be followed by medical or clinical laboratories to ensure generation of quality data and facilitate the acceptance of clinical data by regulatory authorities.

- The bio-analytical laboratories should have SOPs for all activities.

- Two important tools are essential for maintaining laboratory quality: Internal quality control and external quality control.

- Data management system should be in place to ensure timely delivery of high quality data that are necessary to comply with GCP, statistical analysis and reporting. There should be independent data monitoring committee to assess the progress of the study.

# CHAPTER 8

# Bioavailability and Bioequivalence Studies

"In my experience" is a phrase that usually introduces a statement of rank, prejudice or bias. The information that follows it cannot be checked, nor has it been subjected to any analysis other than some vague tally in the speaker's memory.

Michael Crichton, 1971
New England Journal of Medicine

**After reading this chapter, you should be able to:**

- Understand the concept of Bioavailability and Bioequivalence.
- Know when the Bioequivalence testing is necessary.
- Understand the Indian guidelines for Bioequivalence Testing.
- Know how to calculate Bioequivalence from blood level data.

Though the drugs exert their effect by any one of the following methods: through physical action (ointment providing protective effect on skin); by reacting chemically (gastric antacids reducing acidity in the stomach); by modifying the metabolic activity of invading pathogens (antibiotics against bacterial infections); or by modifying the biochemical or metabolic process of body's cells or enzyme systems to change the course of a disease process; the majority of the drugs act by the fourth mechanism (acting on receptors or enzymes). Accordingly the drug development research focuses on this.

Assuming the drug effects through the fourth mechanism, the magnitude of the response is related to the concentration of drug achieved at the site of action. Though this drug concentration depends on several factors like characteristics of drug, dosage form, physiological factors etc., the rate and extent of the entry of the drug to the systemic circulation are determining factors for drug action. The rate and extent at which drug from the administered dosage form appears in the systemic circulation refers as bioavailability (BA). Bioavailability of an active substance from a pharmaceutical product should be known and reproducible from batch to batch.

The same drug when formulated in different dosage forms (and even same dosage forms but formulated differently) may have different bioavailability parameters and thus exhibit different clinical effectiveness. On the other hand, the different products of the same drug, when show similar bioavailability, are likely to produce similar therapeutic effects. When different products (same dosage form) of the same drug show no statistically significant difference in bioavailability among themselves, then they are called bioequivalent.

Studies in bioequivalence (BE) are the commonly accepted method to demonstrate therapeutic equivalence between two medicinal products. Savings in time and costs are substantial when using bioequivalence as an established surrogate marker of therapeutic equivalence. Several test methods are described in order to assess the equivalence (interchangeability): Bioequivalence, comparative pharmacodynamic studies, comparative clinical trials, and *in vitro* dissolution tests.

For all new drug substances and for new dosage forms administered for systemic absorption (which are approved elsewhere in the world), bioequivalence studies with the available formulation should be carried out wherever applicable. Data on the extent of systemic absorption may be required for formulations not meant for systemic absorption. Evaluation of the effect of food on absorption following oral administration should be carried out if the food absorption data is not submitted.

BA/BE (bioequivalence) studies are also clinical studies conducted most often in normal volunteers. Hence, all safeguards to protect participants must be in place, including ethical review of protocol, recruitment methods, compensation for participation, evidence of non-coercion and consent procedures. It is in such studies that the volunteers often participate at short intervals and may participate at different centres within less than the prescribed period of three months between two studies. Mechanisms to prevent this must be developed at the study site.

The Government of India (CDSCO) has developed guidelines for conducting BA/BE studies in India (available from CDSCO website). Though guideline covers the detailed description of BA/BE studies, the present text describes the salient points only for easy understanding by the readers. The readers are encouraged to see full guideline.

BA/BE studies are required to ensure therapeutic equivalence between pharmaceutically equivalent test product and a reference product. For the purpose of establishing bioequivalence, designated reference product containing the same active ingredient as the new drug, identified by DCGI should be used. Designated reference product will normally be the global innovator's product. For subsequent new drug applications in India DCGI may approve another Indian product as designated reference product.

**When Bioequivalence Studies are Necessary:**

**1. *In vivo* Studies:**

In the following conditions, the *in vivo* documentation of equivalence through a bioequivalence study, a comparative clinical pharmacodynamic study, or a comparative clinical trial, is regarded important:

(a) *Oral immediate release drug formulations with systemic action when one or more of the following criteria apply:*
- Indicated for serious conditions requiring assured therapeutic response;
- Narrow therapeutic window/safety margin; steep dose response curve;
- Complicated pharmacokinetics or incomplete absorption or absorption window, nonlinear pharmacokinetics, high pre-systemic or first pass metabolism (more than 70%);
- Unfavorable physicochemical properties: low solubility, instability, meta-stable modifications, poor permeability etc.

- Availability of documented evidence for bioavailability problems related to drug or similar chemical structure or dosage forms;
- Where high ratio of excipients to active ingredient exists.

(b) *Non oral and non parenteral drug formulations designed to act by systemic absorption (transdermal patches, suppositories etc.)*

(c) *Sustained or modified release formulations designed to act by systemic absorption.*

(d) *Fixed – dose combination products with systemic action.*

(e) *Non – solution pharmaceutical products which are for non-systemic use (oral, nasal, ocular, dermal, rectal, vaginal application etc.) and are intended to act without systemic absorption.* In these cases, bioequivalence concept is not suitable and comparative clinical or pharmacodynamic studies are required to prove equivalence. There is a need for drug concentration measurements in order to assess unintended partial absorption.

Bioequivalence documentation is also needed to establish link between:

- Early and late clinical trial formulations.
- Formulations used in clinical trials and stability studies, if different.
- Clinical trial formulations and to be marketed drug products.

In each of the above comparisons, new formulation or new method of manufacture shall be used as test product; and the prior formulation (or respective method of manufacture) is used as reference product.

**2. *In vitro* Studies:**

*In vitro* dissolution testing may be applied for assessing equivalence in the following circumstances:

(a) *Drugs for which the data are available to substantiate all of the following:*

- Highest dose strength is soluble in 250 ml of an aqueous media over the pH range of 1 – 7.5 at 37 °C.
- At least 90% of the administered oral dose is absorbed based on mass balance determination or in comparison to an intravenous reference dose.

- Dissolution rate is more than 80% within 15 minutes at 37 °C using Indian Pharmacopoeia (IP) apparatus 1 at 50 rpm; or IP apparatus 2 at 100 rpm in a volume of 900 ml or less in each of the following media:

  1. 0.1 N hydrochloric acid or artificial gastric juice (without enzymes);
  2. A pH 4.5 buffer;
  3. A pH 6.8 buffer or artificial intestinal juice (without enzymes).

(b) *Different strengths of the drug manufactured by the same manufacturer and all the following criteria are fulfilled:*

  - The qualitative composition between the strengths is essentially same;
  - The ratio of active strength and excipients between the strengths is essentially same. In case of small strength, the ratio between the excipients is same;
  - The method of manufacture is essentially same;
  - An appropriate equivalence study has been performed on at least one of the strengths of the formulation (usually the highest strength, unless a lower strength is chosen for reason of safety);
  - In case of systemic availability, the pharmacokinetics have been shown to be linear over the therapeutic dose range.

*In vitro* dissolution testing may also be suitable to confirm no variation in quality and performance with minor change either in formulation or manufacturing after approval.

### When Bioequivalence Studies are not Necessary:

In the following circumstances the bioequivalence is self evident and thus the bioequivalence study is not necessary:

(a) When the new drugs are to be administered as aqueous injection containing the same active substance(s) in the same concentration and with same excipients as the reference product.

(b) When the new drug is a solution for oral use containing the same active ingredient in same concentration and does not contain excipient which is known to affect the drug absorption.

(c)   When the new drug is a gas.

(d)   When the new drug is given as powder for reconstitution as a solution and the solution meets the criteria as described in (a) or (b).

(e)   When the new drug is an aqueous otic or ophthalmic or topical product containing the same active ingredient in the same concentration and the same excipients in comparable concentration as that of the reference product.

(f)   When the new drug is an aqueous inhalation product or nasal spray to be administered using same or different device as reference product containing the same active substance in the same concentration and with same excipients in comparable concentrations. *Special in vitro testing is required to assess device performance in comparison with reference standard.*

## Design and Conduct of Studies

The studies are divided into two basic types: pharmacokinetic and pharmacodynamic studies.

### (A) Pharmacokinetic Studies:

1. **Study Design:** Typically if two formulations are to be compared, a two – period, two sequence cross over design is the choice with two period of treatment separated by adequate wash out period (equal to or more than five half life of the drug).

   The alternative study designs include the parallel design for very long half life drug or the replicate design for drug with highly variable disposition.

   Single dose studies generally suffice. In some cases a steady state study design is necessary: dose or time dependent pharmacokinetics, modified release products, where problems of sensitivity preclude sufficiently precise plasma concentration measurements after single dose administration or if intra-individual variability in the plasma concentration or disposition precludes the possibility of demonstrating bioequivalence in a reasonably sized single dose study and this variability is reduced at steady state.

2. **Study Population:**

   (a)   **Number of subjects:** The number of subjects required for study should be statistically significant. It usually follows 80/20 rule. The rule says that the study is large enough to provide a 80% probability to detect a 20% difference in average bioavailability.

The number of subjects to be recruited should be sufficient to allow any possible withdrawal or drop outs from the study. However, the minimum number of subjects should not be less than 16 unless justified for ethical reasons.

**(b)** **Selection Criteria for Subjects:** Normally the healthy adult volunteers of either gender are used but care is required in selection to minimize inter and intra individual variation.

While selecting women especially of child bearing potential, it is necessary to get assurance that they are neither pregnant nor likely to be pregnant until completion of the study. This needs to be confirmed by a pregnancy test immediately prior to the first and the last dose. Women taking contraceptive drugs should normally be excluded from study.

If the drug is intended predominantly for elderly patients, the volunteers of 60 years of age or older are preferable. When the drug product is for either gender, attempts should be made to recruit in similar proportion. When the drug has potential hazard for one group of users, the choice must be narrowed down (studies on teratogenic drugs should be conducted only on males).

For drugs where the risk of toxicity or side effects is significant, studies are required to be carried out in patients with concerned diseases rather than the healthy volunteers.

The subjects to be recruited should be screened thoroughly by means of comprehensive medical examination including clinical laboratory tests, an extensive review of medical history including medication history, use of oral contraceptives, alcohol intake, smoking and use of drugs of abuse.

**(c)** **Genetic Phenotyping:** Phenotyping and/or geneotyping of subjects should be considered for exploratory bioavailability studies and all studies using parallel group design. It may also be considered in cross over studies for safety and pharmacokinetic reasons. If a drug is known to be a subject to major genetic polymorphism, studies could be performed in panel of subjects of known phenotype or genotype.

3. **Study Conditions:** Standardization to the study environment, diet, fluid intake, post dosing postures, exercise, sampling schedules etc., is necessary in order to minimize the variability factors. Usually the study subjects are required to abstain from smoking, drinking alcohol, coffee, tea, xanthine containing foods and beverages and fruit juices during the study.

(a) **Selection of Blood Sampling Points/Schedules:** The blood sampling period in single dose trials of an immediate release product should extend to at least three elimination half lives. Sampling should be continued for a sufficient period to ensure that the area extrapolated from the time of last measured concentration to infinite time is only a small percentage (normally less than 20%) of total AUC.

There should be at least three sampling points during the absorption phase, three to four at the projected $T_{max}$ and four points during the elimination phase.

Intervals between successive data/sampling points used to calculate the half-life elimination rate constant should be not longer than the half life of the study drug.

When urinary excretion method is used, for a single dose study it is necessary to collect urine for seven or more half lives.

(b) **Fasting and Fed State Considerations:** Generally, the single dose study should be conducted after an overnight fast (at least 10 hours), with subsequent fast of 4 hours following dosing. For multiple dose fasting state studies, when an evening dose must be given, two hours of fasting before and after the dose is considered acceptable.

However, when it is recommended that the study drug be given with food, or where the dosage form is a modified release product, fed state studies need to be carried out in addition to the fasting state studies. Fed state studies are also required when fasting state studies make assessment of $C_{max}$ and $T_{max}$ difficult.

Studies in the fed state require the consumption of a high fat breakfast before dosing. It must be consumed approximately 15 minutes before the dosing. Such a breakfast should be designed to provide 950 to 1000 KCals. At least 50% of these calories must come from fat, 15-20% from proteins and the rest from carbohydrates.

**(c) Steady State Studies:** In the following cases, an additional steady state is appropriate:

- When the drug has a long terminal elimination half life and blood concentrations after a single dose cannot be followed for a sufficient time.
- Where assay sensitivity is inadequate to follow the terminal elimination phase for an adequate period of time.
- For toxic drugs which are required to be administered only to patients (not healthy volunteers) and requiring multiple dose therapy (cytotoxics).
- For modified release products where it is necessary to assess the fluctuation in plasma concentration over dosage interval at steady state.
- For those drugs which induce their own metabolism or show large intra-individual variability.
- For enteric coated preparations where the coating is innovative.
- For combination products where the ratio of plasma concentration of the individual drugs is important.
- For drugs that exhibit non-linear (dose or time dependent) pharmacokinetics.
- Where the drug is likely to accumulate in the body.

In steady state studies, the dosing schedule should follow the clinically recommended dosage regimen.

**(d) Characteristics to be investigated:** In most cases, the evaluation of BA and BE is based on the measurement of active drug concentration in biological matrix. In the following cases, the measurement of an active or inactive metabolite may be necessary: (a) where the concentration of the drug may be too low to accurately measure, (b) limitation of analytical method, (c). unstable drug, (d). drug with a short half life, or (e). in case of prodrugs.

Measurement of individual enantiomers using an achiral assay method is recommended where all the following criteria are met:

- The enantiomers exhibit different pharmacodynamic characteristics.
- The enantiomers exhibit different pharmacokinetic characteristics.
- Primary efficacy or safety activities reside with minor enantiomers.
- Non-linear absorption is present for at least one enantiomer.

For assessing the rate and extent of absorption from plasma - time concentration curve the following pharmacokinetic parameters are required to be measured: $C_{max}$, $T_{max}$, $AUC_{0-t}$ and $AUC_{0-\infty}$. For steady state studies, $AUC_{0-\tau}$, $C_{max}$, $C_{min}$ and degree of fluctuation should be calculated.

(e) **Bioanalytical Methodology:** Well characterized, standardized, validated bioanalytical methods should be used. The validation of analytical method can be envisaged to consist of two distinct phases:

- Pre-study phase: It involves the validation of the method on biological matrix: human plasma samples and spiked plasma samples.
- Study phase: The validated analytical method is applied to the actual analysis of samples from bioavailability and bioequivalence studies to confirm the stability, accuracy and precision.

*Pre – Study phase:* The following characteristics of the bioanalytical method must be evaluated and documented to ensure the acceptability of the performance and reliability of the analytical results:

- Stability of the drug or metabolites in the biological matrix: The stability of drug or active metabolites in the biological matrix under the condition of the experiment (including the period of storage) should be established. The stability data should include at least three freezing and thawing cycle representative of actual sample handling. The absence of any sorption by the sampling containers and stoppers should also be established.

- Specificity/Selectivity: Data should be generated to demonstrate that the assay method does not suffer from interference by endogenous compounds, degradation products, other drugs likely to be present in study samples, and metabolites of the drug(s) under study.

- Sensitivity: It is the capacity of the test procedure to record small variations in concentration. The analytical method should be capable of assaying the drug/metabolites over the expected concentration range. A reliable lowest limit of quantification should be established based on intra- and inter-day coefficient of variation usually not greater than 20%. The limit of detection (the lowest concentration that can be differentiated from background levels) is usually lower than the limit of quantification.

- Precision and Accuracy: Precision (the degree of reproducibility of individual assays) should be established by replicate assays on standards, preferably at several concentrations. Accuracy is the degree to which the 'true' value of the concentration of the drug is estimated by the assay. Precision and accuracy should normally be documented at three concentrations (low, medium, high) where 'low' is the vicinity of the lowest concentration to be measured, 'high' is a value in the vicinity of $C_{max}$ and 'medium' is a suitable intermediate value.

Intra – assay precision (within days) in terms of coefficient of variation should be no more than 15%, although no more than 20% may be more realistic at values near the lower limit of quantification. Inter – assay precision (between days) may be higher than 15% but not more than 20%.

In general the accuracy of ± 15% should be attained.

- Recovery: Documentation of extraction recovery at high, medium and low concentrations is essential. If the recovery is low, alternative method should be explored. Low recoveries are more prone to inconsistency. Recovery of any internal standard used should also be investigated.

- Range and Linearity: The quantitative relationship between concentration and response should be adequately characterized over the entire range of expected sample concentrations. The standard curve should be defined by at least five concentrations.

If the concentration – response function is non-linear, additional points would be necessary to define the non-linear portions of the curve. Extrapolation beyond the standard curve is not acceptable.

- Analytical System Stability: To ensure that the analytical system remains stable over the time course of the assay, the reproducibility of the standard curve should be monitored during the assay.

***Study Phase:*** In general, the analysis of biological samples can be done by single determination without a need for duplicate or replicate analysis. The need for duplicate analysis should be assessed on case by case.

A standard curve should be generated for each analytical run for each analyte and should be used to calculate the concentration of the analyte in the unknown samples assayed with the run. Standard curve should cover the entire range of concentrations in the unknown samples. Estimation of unknown by extrapolation of standard curve below the lowest standard concentration or above the highest standard concentration is not recommended. It is suggested that the standard curve should be re-determined or samples should be re-assayed after dilution. Quality control sample should be used to accept or reject the run.

***Quality Control Samples:*** They are samples with known concentration prepared by spiking drug free biological fluid with the drug. These samples should be prepared in low, medium and high concentrations.

To avoid possible confusion between quality control samples and standard solutions during the review process, preparation of quality control samples at concentrations different from those used for calibration is recommended. For stable analytes, quality control samples should be prepared in the fluid of interest at the time of the pre study assay validation or at the time of study sample collection, and stored with the study samples. For less stable analytes, daily or weekly quality control samples may have to be prepared.

A quality control sample for each concentration should be assayed on each occasion that the study samples are assayed, and the concentration determined by reference to that day's calibration standards. If the concentration values determined for the controls are not within ±15% of the expected concentrations, the batch should be considered for re-analysis.

***Repeat Analysis:*** Aberrant results due to processing errors, equipments failure, or poor chromatography demands re-analysis of samples. The reasons for re-analysis must be stated. The criteria for repeat analysis should be determined prior to running study and recorded in the protocol of laboratory SOP.

**(f) Statistical Evaluation:**

    **(i) Data Analysis:** Appropriate statistical methods for data analysis and adequate sample size should be used to limit the consumer's risk (erroneously accepting bio-equivalence) and minimizing the manufacturer's risk as well (erroneously rejecting bioequivalence).

    **(ii) Statistical Analysis:** The statistical analysis (ANOVA) should take into account the sources of variation that can be reasonably assumed to have an effect on the response. The 90% confidence interval for the ratio of population means (test/reference) or two one sided - t tests with the full hypothesis of non bioequivalence at the 5% significance level for the parameter under consideration are considered for testing bioequivalence.

    Logarithmic transformation of the data ($C_{max}$ and AUC) should be carried out before performing statistical analysis. The analysis of $T_{max}$ is desirable if it is clinically significant. The parameter $T_{max}$ should be analyzed using non-parametric methods.

(iii) **Criteria for Bioequivalence:** The calculated 90% confidence interval for AUC and $C_{max}$ should fall within 80-125% bioequivalence range. This is equivalent to the rejection of two one sided – t tests with the null hypothesis of non-bioequivalence at 5% level of significance. The non-parametric 90% confidence interval for $T_{max}$ should lie within a clinically acceptable range.

Tighter limits for permissible difference in bioavailability may be required for drugs that have:

- Narrow therapeutic index.
- Serious dose related toxicity.
- Steep dose/effect curve, or a non-linear pharmacokinetics within the therapeutic range.

A wider acceptance range may be acceptable if it is based on sound clinical justification.

In case of supra-bioavailability (test product has much more bioavailability than reference product), a reformulation followed by a fresh bioavailability testing may be necessary. Such formulations are usually not acceptable as therapeutic equivalent.

(iv) **Deviation from the study plan:** The method of analysis should be defined in the protocol. The protocol should specify methods for handling drop outs and for identifying biologically implausible outliers. A scientific explanation should be provided to justify the exclusion of a volunteer from the analysis.

(g) **Special Considerations for Modified Release Products:** The modified release products means: delayed release, sustained release, mixed immediate and sustained release, mixed delayed and sustained release and mixed immediate and delayed release.

Generally these products should:

- Act as modified release formulations and meet the label claim.
- Preclude the possibility of any dose dumping effect.
- There must be significant difference between the performance of modified release products and the conventional release product.
- Provide a therapeutic performance comparable to the reference immediate release formulation administered by the same route in multiple doses (of an equivalent daily amount) or to the reference modified release formulation.
- Produce consistent pharmacokinetic performance between individual dosage units, and
- Produce plasma levels which lie within the therapeutic range for the proposed dosing intervals at steady state.

If all the above conditions are not met, sufficient justification is to be given to make the product acceptable.

***Study Parameters***: Bioavailability data should be obtained for all modified release products. If the formulation is the first market entry of the drug substance, the product's pharmacokinetic parameters should be determined. If the formulation is a second or subsequent market entry, then comparative bioavailability studies using an appropriate reference standard should be performed.

***Study Design***: Single dose or single and multiple dose study are to be conducted both in fasted and non fasting state. If the effect of food on the reference product is not known, two separate two way cross over studies: one in fasted state and the other in fed state may be carried out. If it is known with certainty that food affect reference product (from published data), then a three – way cross over study may be appropriate with:

- Reference product in the fasting state,
- Test product in the fasted state, and
- Test product in fed state.

***Requirements for modified release formulations unlikely to accumulate:*** The dosing interval is such that it is not likely to lead to accumulation in the body ($AUC_{0-\tau}$ /$AUC_{0-\infty} \geq 0.8$).

When the modified release product is the first market entry of that type of dosage from, the reference product is the innovator's immediate release formulation. The comparison should be between a single dose of the modified release formulation and doses of immediate release formulation which it intends to replace. The latter must be administered according to the established dosing regimen.

When the modified release product is the second or subsequent entry on the market, comparison is to be made with the reference modified release product for which bioequivalence is claimed.

Studies should be performed with single dose administration in the fasting state as well as following an appropriate meal at a specified time. The following parameters are to be determined from plasma (or, other relevant biological fluid) concentrations of the drug and

or major metabolites: $AUC_{0-\tau}$ , $AUC_{0-t}$, $AUC_{0-\infty}$ and $C_{max}$ and $K_{el}$.

The 90% confidence interval calculated using log transformed data for the ratios (test : reference) of the geometric mean AUC (for both $AUC_{0-\tau}$ and $AUC_{0-t}$) and $C_{max}$ (where the comparison is with an existing modified release product) should generally be within the range 80 to 125% both in the fasting state and following the administration of an appropriate meal at a specified time before taking the drug.

***Requirements for modified release formulations likely to accumulate:*** The dosing interval is such that it is likely to lead to accumulation ($AUC_{0-\tau}$ /$AUC_{0-\infty} \leq 0.8$).

When the modified release product is the first market entry of that type of dosage from, the reference product is the innovator's immediate release formulation. Both a single dose and steady state doses of the modified release formulation should be compared with doses of immediate-release formulation which it is intended to replace. The latter must be administered according to the established dosing regimen.

Studies should be performed with single dose administration in the fasting state as well as following an appropriate meal. In addition, studies are required at steady state. For single dose studies, the following pharmacokinetic parameters are to be determined: $AUC_{0-\tau}$, $AUC_{0-t}$, $AUC_{0-\infty}$, $C_{max}$ and $K_{el}$.

For steady state studies the following parameters: $AUC_{0-\tau\ (ss)}$, $C_{max}$, $C_{min}$, and $C_{pd}$ and degree of fluctuation are to be determined.

When the modified release product is the second or subsequent entry on the market, single dose and steady sate comparison is to be made with the reference modified release product for which bioequivalence is claimed.

The 90% confidence interval for the ratio of geometric means (test:reference) of AUC (for both $AUC_{0-\tau}$ and $AUC_{0-t}$) and $C_{max}$ (where the comparison is with an existing modified release product) determined using log transformed data should generally be within the range 80 to 125% when the products are compared after single dose administration in both the fasting state and fed state.

The 90% confidence interval for the ratio of geometric means (test:reference) for $AUC_{0-\tau\ (ss)}$, $C_{max}$ and $C_{min}$ determined using log –transformed data should generally be within the range 80 – 125% when the formulations are compared at steady state.

When these studies do not show bioequivalence, comparative efficacy and safety data may be required for the new product.

**(B) Pharmacodynamic Studies:** The pharmacodynamic studies for establishing equivalence between two pharmaceutical products may be required if quantitative analysis of the drug and /or metabolite(s) in plasma or urine cannot be made with sufficient accuracy and sensitivity. Further, these studies are required if measurements of drug concentrations cannot be used as surrogate end points for demonstration of efficacy and safety of the particular pharmaceutical product like topical products without an intended absorption of the drug into the systemic circulation. For details, the readers are encouraged to see the original guidelines issued by CDSCO.

**(C) Comparative Clinical Studies:** This type of study is required when pharmacokinetic and pharmacodynamic studies are not feasible. For details, the readers are encouraged to see the original guidelines issued by CDSCO.

**(D) *In Vitro* Studies:** Earlier it is discussed about the situations where a comparative *in vitro* study may be sufficient to demonstrate equivalence between two drug products.

The test methodology adopted should be in line with Pharmacopoeial requirements unless those requirements are shown to be unsatisfactory. Dissolution studies should generally be carried out under mild agitation conditions at 37±0.5 °C and at physiologically relevant pH. More than one batch of each formulation should be tested. Comparative dissolution profiles, rather than single point dissolution test data, should be generated. The design should include:

- Individually testing of at least 12 dosage units (tablets/capsules etc) of each batch. Mean and individual results should be reported along with their standard deviations or standard errors.

- Measuring the percentage of nominal content released at a number of suitably spaced time points to provide a profile for each batch (at 10, 20 and 30 minutes or as appropriate)    to achieve virtually complete dissolution.

- Determining the dissolution profile in at least three aqueous media covering the pH range of 1.0 to 6.8 or in cases where it is considered necessary, pH range of 1.0 to 8.0.

- Conducting the tests on each batch using the same apparatus and, if possible, on the same or consecutive days.

Comparison of dissolution profiles may be done by any of the established models : independent or model - dependent methods.

**Documentation:**

The following important documents must be maintained:

(i)   Clinical data:
   (a) All relevant documents as required to be maintained for compliance with GCP guidelines.

   (ii)  Details of analytical method validation including the following:

     (a)  System suitability test.

     (b)  Linear range.

     (c)  Lowest limit of quantification.

     (d)  QC sample analysis.

     (e)  Stability sample analysis.

     (f)  Recovery experiment result.

  (iii)  Analytical data of volunteer plasma samples which should include the following:

     (a)  Validation data of analytical methods used.

     (b)  Chromatograms of all volunteers, including any aberrant chromatograms.

     (c)  Inter-day and intra-day variation of assay results.

     (d)  Details including chromatograms of any repeat analysis performed.

     (e)  Calibration status of the instruments.

  (iv)  Raw data.

  (v)  All comments of the chief investigator regarding the data of the study submitted for review.

  (vi)  A copy of the final report.

***Study Report:*** The bioequivalence or bioavailability report should give the complete documentation of its protocol, conduct and evaluation.

The report should include (as a minimum) the following information:

  (a)  Table of contents.

  (b)  Title of the study.

  (c)  Names and credentials of responsible investigators.

  (d)  Signatures of the principal and other responsible investigators authenticating their respective sections of the report.

  (e)  Site of the study and facilities used.

  (f)  The period of dates over which the clinical and analytical steps were conducted.

(g) Names and batch numbers of products compared.

(h) A signed declaration that this was identical to that intended for marketing.

(i) Results of assays and other pharmaceutical tests (e.g., physical description, dimensions, mean weight, weight uniformity, and comparative dissolution) carried out on the batches of products compared.

(j) Full protocol for the study including a copy of the ICF and criteria for inclusion/exclusion or withdrawal of subjects.

(k) Report of protocol deviations, violations.

(l) Documentary evidence that the study was approved by an independent ethics committee and was carried out in accordance with GCP/GLP.

(m) Demographic data of subjects.

(n) Details names and addresses of the subjects.

(o) Details of and justifications of protocol deviations.

(p) Details of drop out and withdrawals from the study should be fully documented and accounted for.

(q) Details of analytical methods used, full validation data, quality control data and criteria for accepting or rejecting assay results.

(r) Representative chromatograms covering the whole concentration range for all, standard and quality control samples as well as specimens analyzed.

(s) Sampling schedules and deviations of the actual times from the scheduled.

(t) Details of how pharmacokinetic parameters were calculated.

(u) Documentation related to statistical analysis:

    (i) Randomization schedule.

    (ii) Volunteer wise plasma concentration and time points for test and reference products.

    (iii) Volunteer wise $AUC_{0-t}$, $AUC_{0-\infty}$, $C_{max}$, $T_{max}$, $K_{el}$, and $t_{1/2}$ for test and reference products.

    (iv) Logarithmic transformed measures used for BE demonstration.

(v)   ANOVA for $AUC_{0-t}$, $AUC_{0-\infty}$, $C_{max}$.

(vi)  Inter-subject, intra-subject and /or total variability if possible.

(vii) Confidence Intervals (CI) for $AUC_{0-t}$, $AUC_{0-\infty}$, $C_{max}$ (Confidence Interval values should not be rounded off): to pass a CI range of 80 to 125, the values should be at least 80.00 and not more than 125.00.

(viii) Geometric mean, arithmetic mean, ratio of means for $AUC_{0-t}$, $AUC_{0-\infty}$, $C_{max}$.

(ix)  Partial AUC, only if it is used.

(x)   $C_{min}$, $C_{max}$, $AUC_{0-\tau}$, degree of fluctuation $[(C_{max} - C_{min})/C_{av}]$ and swing $[(C_{max} - C_{min})/C_{min}]$, if steady state studies are employed.

## Facilities Required for BA and BE Studies

(a) **Legal Identity:** The organization, conducting BA/BE studies, or the parent organization to which it belongs, must be a legally constituted body with appropriate statutory registrations.

(b) **Impartiality, Confidentiality, Independence and Integrity:** The organization shall:

- Have managerial staff with authority and the resources needed to discharge their duties.

- Have arrangements to ensure that its personnel are free from any commercial, financial and other pressures which might adversely affect the quality of their work.

- Be organized in such a way that the confidence in its independence of judgment and integrity is maintained at all times.

- Have documented policies and procedures, where relevant, to ensure the protection of its sponsors' confidential information and proprietary rights.

- Not engage in any activity that may jeopardize the trust in its independence of judgment and integrity.

- Have documented policies and procedures for the safety of human subjects and the use of human subjects in research is consistence with Schedule Y of Drugs and Cosmetics Rules and GCP guidelines.

- Have documented policies and procedures for scientific integrity including procedures dealing with and reporting possible scientific misconduct.

**(c) Organization and Management:** The study site organization must include the following:

(i) Any investigator who has the overall responsibility to provide medical care to the human subjects. The investigator(s) should possess appropriate medical qualifications and relevant experience for conducting pharmacokinetic studies.

(ii) The site should have identified adequately qualified and trained personnel to perform the following functions:

- Clinical Pharmacological Unit (CPU) management.
- Analytical laboratory management.
- Data handling and interpretation.
- Documentation and report preparation.
- Quality assurance of all operations in the centre.

**(d) Documented Standard Operating Procedures:** The centre should establish and maintain a quality system appropriate to the type, range and volume of its activities. All operations at the site must be conducted as per authorized and documented standard operating procedures (SOPs). These documented procedures should be available to the respective personnel for ready reference. The procedures covered must include those that ensure compliance with all aspects of GCP Guidelines and Good Laboratory Practice (GLP) guidelines issued by Ministry of Health and Family Welfare.

A partial list of procedures for which documented SOPs should be made available includes:

(i) Maintenance of working standards (pure substances) and respective documentation.

(ii) Withdrawal, storage, and handling of biological samples.

(iii) Maintenance, calibration and validation of instruments.

(iv) Managing medical as well as non-medical emergency situations.

(v) Handling of biological fluids.

(vi) Managing laboratory hazards.

(vii) Procedure for disposal of clinical samples and laboratory wastes.

(viii) Documentation of clinical pharmacology unit observations, volunteer data and analytical data.

(ix) Obtaining informed consent from volunteers.

(x) Volunteer screening and recruitment and management of ineligible volunteers.

(xi) Randomization code management.

(xii) Study subject management at the site (including check-in and check-out procedures).

(xiii) Recording and reporting protocol deviations.

(xiv) Recording, reporting and managing scientific misconduct.

(xv) Monitoring and quality assurance.

Wherever possible, disposable (sterile, wherever applicable) medical devices must be used for making subject interventions.

If services of a laboratory or a facility other than those available at the site (whether within India or outside the country) are to be availed, its/their name(s), address(s) and specific services to be used should be documented.

(e) **Clinical Pharmacological Unit:** The unit must have adequate space and facilities to house at least 16 volunteers. Adequate area must be provided for dining and recreation of volunteers, separate from their sleeping area.

Additional space and facilities should also be provided for the following:

(i) Office and administrative functions

(ii) Sample Collection and storage

(iii) Control sample storage

(iv) Wet chemical laboratory

(v) Instrumental Laboratory

(vi) Library

(vii) Documentation archival room

(viii) Facility for washing, cleaning and Toilets

(ix) Microbiological laboratory (Optional)

(x) Radio Immuno - Assay room (optional)

## Maintenance of Records of BA/BE Studies

All records of *in vivo* and *in vitro* tests conducted on any marketed batch of a drug product to assure that the product meets a bioequivalence requirement shall be maintained by the sponsor for at least 2 years after expiration date of the batch and submitted to CDSCO on request.

## Retention of BA/BE Samples

All samples of test and reference drug products used in bioavailability / bioequivalence study should be retained for a period of three years after the conduct of the study or one year after the expiry of the drug, which ever is earlier. The study sponsor and /or drug manufacturer should provide the testing facility batches and the reference drug products in such a manner that the reserve samples can be selected randomly. This is to ensure that the samples are infact the representative of the batches and they are retained in their original containers. Each reserve sample should have adequate quantity to carry out twice all the *in vitro* and *in vivo* tests required during BA/BE study.

The reserve sample should be stored in consistence with product labeling and in an area segregated from the area where testing is conducted and with access limited to authorized personnel.

## Special Topics

(a) **Food Effect Bioavailability Studies:** Food effect study is required when there is a possibility to have effect of food on the bioavailability of the drug. Food effect bioavailability studies focus on effects of food on the release of the drug substance from the drug product as well as the absorption of drug substance. Usually a single dose cross over study is recommended for BA and BE studies.

(b) **Long half-life drugs:** For BE determination of an oral product with long half life, a single dose cross over study can be conducted, provided an adequate wash out period is used. If due to longer periods, chances of drop outs as well as intra subject variation are higher with routine cross over designs; parallel group designs can be used. In all cases, blood sampling period should be adequate to describe the plasma concentration time profile. $C_{max}$ and a suitably truncated AUC can be used to characterize peak and total drug exposure, respectively. For drugs, demonstrating high intra-subject variability in distribution and clearance, AUC truncation warrants caution. In such cases, sponsors and/or applicants should consult the regulatory authority.

(c) **Early Exposure:** In general, bioequivalence may be demonstrated by measurements of peak and total exposure for an immediate release product. However, in situations such as rapid onset of an analgesic effect or to avoid an excessive hypotensive action of an antihypertensive, an early exposure measure may be informative on the basis of appropriate clinical efficacy/safety trials and /or pharmacokinetic / pharmacodynamic studies that call for better control of drug absorption into the systemic circulation. In these situations, use of partial AUC is recommended as an early exposure measure. The partial area should be truncated at $T_{max}$ values for the reference formulation. Atleast two quantifiable samples should be collected before the expected peak time, to allow adequate estimation of the partial area.

(d) **Individual and Population Bioequivalence:** The current practice of evaluating BE has been termed as "average bioequivalence". Whereas in individual BE, determination of intra-subject variation of drug response is important. By "population BE", it is meant a bioequivalence criterion that requires the distribution of the formulation to be sufficiently similar to that of reference in some appropriate population. Average BE is a special case of population BE.

The average BE of two formulations is important in the case of prescribability. However, individual bioequivalence is required incase of switchability.

Assessment of individual BE is an interesting and exciting alternative to the current practice of evaluating average BE. The evaluation of individual BE requires values of intra-subject variability of the test and reference formulations. Hence, the assessment of individual BE is done based on three or four period designs. Replicate study designs provide such information.

Until now, BE studies are designed to evaluate average BE. Experience with population and individual BE studies is limited. Hence no specific recommendation is proposed on this matter. However, for highly variable drugs, individual BE can be considered.

# Documents to be Submitted for Grant of Permission to Conduct Bioequivalence Studies for Export Purpose

**(I) Requirements for BE study of a new molecule not approved in India but approved in the other countries.**

1. Application in Form-44 (Drugs and Cosmetics Act and the Rules) duly signed, by the competent authority with name and designation.

2. Treasury Challan of Rs. 25000/- as per Drugs & Cosmetic Rules.

3. Undertaking by the Principal Investigator (PI) as per appendix VII of schedule "Y" of Drugs and Cosmetic Rules.

4. A copy of the approval granted to the BE study centre by CDSCO.

5. Sponsor's authorization letter duly signed by the competent authority on their letterhead.

6. The study protocols.

7. The study synopsis.

8. Pre-clinical single dose data and repeated dose toxicity data.

9. Clinical study data and published report of pharmacokinetic and pharmacodynamic study carried out in healthy volunteers/patients data published in reputed journals.

10. Regulatory status of the drug.

11. Names of the countries where the drug is currently being marketed (to be mentioned in the covering letter also).

12. Package literature on the international product.

13. Complete Certificate of Analysis of same batches (both test & reference formulations) to be used in the BE study.

14. In the case of multiple dose BE study, adequate supporting safety data should be submitted.

15. In the case of Injectable preparation, the sub-acute toxicity data should be submitted on the product, generated in two species for adequate duration.

16. Depending on the nature of the drug like cytoxic agent, hormonal preparations etc. Proper justification for conducting studies on healthy volunteers/patients or male/ female should be submitted.

## (II) New Drugs approved in India within period of 1 year

1. Application in Form-44 (Drugs and Cosmetics Act and the Rules) duly signed, by the competent authority with name and designation.

2. Treasury Challan of Rs. 25000/- as per Drugs & Cosmetic Rules.

3. Undertaking by the Principal Investigator (PI) as per appendix VII of schedule "Y" of Drugs and Cosmetic Rules.

4. A copy of the approval of the BE study centre from CDSCO.

5. Sponsor's authorization letter duly signed by the competent authority on their letterhead.

6. The study protocols.

7. Clinical study data and published report of pharmacokinetic and pharmacodynamic study carried out in healthy volunteers data published in reputed journals.

8. Package literature on the international product.

9. Complete Certificate of Analysis of same batches (both test & reference formulations) to be used in the BE study.

10. In the case of multiple dose BE study adequate supporting safety data should be submitted.

11. In the case of injectable preparation, the sub-acute toxicity data should be submitted on the product, generated in two species for adequate duration.

12. Depending on the nature of the drug like cytoxic agent, hormonal preparations etc. Proper justification for conducting studies on healthy volunteers/patients or male/ female should be submitted.

## (III) New drugs approved within period of more than 1 year & less than 4 years

1. Application in Form-44 duly signed, by the competent authority with name and designation.

2. Treasury Challan of Rs. 15000/- as per Drugs & Cosmetic Rules.

3. Undertaking by the Principal Investigator (PI) as per appendix VII of schedule "Y" of Drugs and Cosmetic Rules.

4. A copy of the approval of the BE study centre from CDSCO.

5. Sponsor's authorization letter duly signed on their letterhead by the competent authority.

6. The study protocols.

7. Complete Certificate of Analysis of same batches (both test & reference formulations) to be used in the BE study.

8. In the case of multiple dose BE study, adequate supporting safety data should be submitted.

9. In the case of Injectable preparation, the sub-acute toxicity data should be submitted on the product, generated in two species for adequate duration.

10. Depending on the nature of the drug like cytoxic agent, hormonal preparations etc. Proper justification for conducting studies on healthy volunteers/patients or male/ female should be submitted.

**(IV) BE NOC for all the drug products in modified release form irrespective of their approval status**

1. Application in Form-44 (Drugs and Cosmetics Act and the Rules) duly signed, by the competent authority with name and designation.

2. Treasury Challan of Rs. 15000/- as per Drugs & Cosmetic Rules.

3. Undertaking by the Principal Investigator (PI) as per appendix VII of schedule "Y" of Drugs and Cosmetic Rules.

4. A copy of the approval of the BE study centre from CDSCO.

5. Sponsor's authorization letter duly signed on their letterhead by the competent authority.

6. The study protocols.

7. Complete Certificate of Analysis of same batches (both test & reference formulations) to be used in the BE study.

8. In the case of multiple dose BE study, adequate supporting safety data should be submitted.

9. In the case of Injectable preparation, the sub-acute toxicity data should be submitted on the product generated data in two species for adequate duration.

10. Depending on the nature of the drug like cytoxic agent, hormonal preparations etc. Proper justification for conducting studies on healthy volunteers/patients or male/ female should be submitted.

All the above requirements are general in nature, however depending on the nature of the drug, disease and studies further specific information may also be required to be furnished by the firm.

***Bioequivalence Testing***: Simple Exercise to give preliminary knowledge on how the testing is conducted. Readers are encouraged to look at more details in Pharmaceutical Statistics book. Only one parameter (AUC) is calculated. Other parameters like $C_{max}$ and $T_{max}$ should also be calculated similarly.

| Subject | $AUC_{test}$ (µg. h/ml) | log $AUC_{test}$ | $AUC_{reference}$ (µg. h/ml) | log $AUC_{referenc}$ | log difference |
|---|---|---|---|---|---|
| 1 | 120.9 | 2.082 | 149.4 | 2.174 | -0.092 |
| 2 | 166.7 | 2.221 | 132.1 | 2.120 | 0.101 |
| 3 | 150.1 | 2.176 | 139.8 | 2.145 | 0.031 |
| 4 | 108.7 | 2.036 | 179.1 | 2.253 | -0.217 |
| 5 | 184.2 | 2.265 | 162.1 | 2.209 | 0.056 |
| 6 | 134.1 | 2.127 | 135.3 | 2.131 | -0.004 |
| 7 | 227.5 | 2.356 | 132.5 | 2.122 | 0.234 |
| 8 | 145.6 | 2.163 | 121.5 | 2.084 | 0.079 |
| 9 | 153.2 | 2.185 | 131.5 | 2.118 | 0.067 |
| 10 | 259.2 | 2.413 | 160.6 | 2.205 | 0.208 |
| 11 | 127.8 | 2.106 | 177.0 | 2.247 | -0.141 |
| 12 | 187.3 | 2.272 | 193.7 | 2.287 | -0.015 |
| Average (mean) | | | | | 0.0255 |
| Standard Deviation (SD) | | | | | 0.1317 |

For 90% confidence interval, the value of t from t table for 11 degree of freedom = 1.796

The High and low bound confidence interval can be obtained from the equation:

Antilog of $\text{Mean} \pm \dfrac{SD \times t\,value}{\sqrt{N}}$ where t value is obtained from t table for required confidence interval and degree of freedom; N = Number of subjects.

High Bound Confidence Interval = Antilog of $(\text{Mean} + \dfrac{SD \times t\,value}{\sqrt{N}}) =$

Antilog of $( 0.0255 + \dfrac{0.1317 \times 1.796}{\sqrt{12}} = 1.24 );$

Low Bound Confidence Interval = Antilog of $(\text{Mean} - \dfrac{SD \times t\,value}{\sqrt{N}}) =$

Antilog of $(0.0255 - \dfrac{0.1317 \times 1.796}{\sqrt{12}}) = 1.06$

To establish bioequivalence, the calculated confidence interval should fall within a bioequivalence limit, usually 80-125% for the ratio of the product averages (i.e. 0.80 – 1.25).

In this AUC comparison, the calculated confidence interval range is 1.06 to 1.24 which indicates that it is within the range of 0.80 to 1.25.

Thus in terms of AUC, the test product is bioequivalent to reference product.

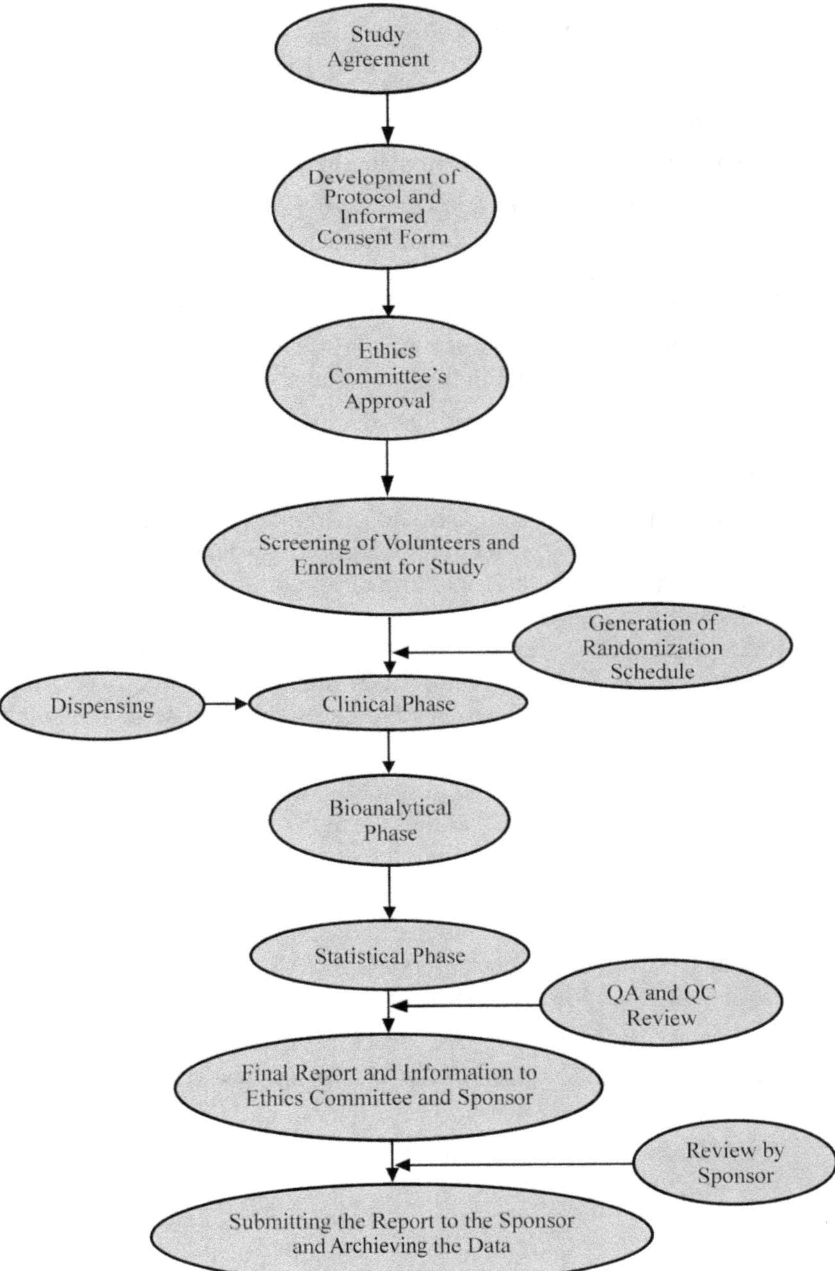



**Fig. 8.1** Typical Flow Chart of Bioequivalence Study in a CRO.

## Key Points to Remember

- The rate and extent of entry of the drug to the systemic circulation are determining factors for drug action. The rate and extent at which drug from the administered dosage form appears in the systemic circulation is called bioavailability.

- When different products (same dosage forms) of the same drug show no statistically significant difference in bioavailability among themselves, then they are called bioequivalent. Bioequivalent products are therapeutic equivalent and are interchangeable.

- Bioavailability or Bioequivalence (BA/BE) studies are clinical studies usually conducted in healthy human volunteers.

- Bioequivalency may be established either through *in vivo* or *in vitro* studies. The *in vivo* studies are usually necessary in the following situations: oral immediate release drug formulations with systemic action; non oral and non-parenteral drug formulations designed to act by systemic absorption; sustained or modified release formulations designed to act by systemic absorption; and fixed dose combinations with systemic action. For non-solution products for non-systemic use, BE concept is not applicable but comparative clinical and pharmacodynamic studies are necessary. The *in vitro* dissolution testing may be used to assess equivalency when the drug is highly soluble in water.

- BE studies may be of pharmacokinetics or pharmacodynamic types. Pharmacokinetic studies should be conducted with appropriate study design keeping the conditions of the study for the test and reference product similar.

- $C_{max}$, $T_{max}$ and AUC are the parameters for assessing BE. The calculated 90% confidence interval for AUC and $C_{max}$ should fall within 80-125% bioequivalence range.

- Pharmacodynamic studies are necessary when measurement of drug or metabolite concentration cannot be made with sufficient accuracy and sensitivity.

- BE studies should be conducted after obtaining regulatory approval and following GCP.

# CHAPTER 9

# Data Management in Clinical Research

"With integrity, you have nothing to fear, since you have nothing to hide.
With integrity, you will do the right thing, so you will have no guilt."

ZigZiglar

**After reading this chapter, you should be able to understand:**
- What are data and their importance in clinical research;
- Roles and responsibilities of clinical data management persons;
- Principles of Good Data Management Practices; and
- Tools available for data management.

The clinical trial is a fundamental step in drug discovery & development and is linked to the robustness and accuracy of data submitted by the sponsor to the drug regulatory authority. The clinical trials generate data which are analyzed to either prove or disprove a research hypothesis. The usual hypothesis is 'benefits outweigh the risks'. The data must be comprehensive, complete, accurate and true to assure the quality of studies. This is a question of trust and belief. The healthcare decisions for a treatment are based on the data generated during clinical research. Evidence based medicines are practiced based on these data. Clinical trials being the very expensive process, it cannot afford to have unreliable results and it is necessary to have procedures to reduce slippage in the process.

The 'data' may be defined as factual information (as measurements or statistics) used as a basis for reasoning, discussion or calculation. In other words, data are any information or observations that are associated with a particular research including experimental specimens, technologies and products related to research. The examples of data are: patient survey response, temperature readings, metabolism rates, patient's symptoms, population health habits.

Thus, data are not just information or observations but also includes materials, products, procedures, and other data sources that are part of the research project.

There has been the cause of concern as the clinical research data are under scanner and many clinical research organizations received warning letters from the overseas regulatory authorities. The readers can find few press reports described later in text box. Unreliable or falsified data not only causes dis-reputation but also leads to patients' injury. The 'data integrity' may be defined as "maintaining and assuring the accuracy and consistency of the data over the entire life cycle".

**Clinical Data Management Systems:** The clinical trials generate increasing amount of data, as required by the regulatory authorities, which must be collected, processed and analyzed. This requires a system often called Clinical Data Management System (CDMS). Thus, CDM is defined as the process of collection, cleaning, and management of subject data in compliance with regulatory standards. The primary objective of CDM processes is to provide high-quality data by keeping the number of errors and missing data as low as possible and gather maximum data for analysis. Even if several tools including software are advocated for data management, there are several issues in data management. In short, CDMS is the tool for clinical data management.

The data may be obtained through remote capturing or directly from clinical trial sites using remote data capture or using more paper based method. There must be a clinical data management team whose responsibility is to keep the project team including sponsor on the status of the project on ongoing basis. It is necessary to have tailor made on ongoing made information to meet the requirements of sponsor and other stake holders. This should help the sponsor to know what has happened in the study, what is happening and what is going to happen:

- Frequency of report: Preferably weekly to sponsor (pertaining to new progress that have happened after the last report). Monthly or bimonthly reporting is also practiced.
- Format: Simple Microsoft excel spread to hyper linking of files.
- Method: E-mailing is preferable.

The clinical data management process usually begins with the establishment of data management group and ends with delivery of quality database. The database must be accurate, secure, reliable and ready for analysis. The process activities are:

I. **Development of data management plan (DMP):** The DMP is study specific and should be made in the beginning of the study. It is a living document throughout the life cycle of the study and should have scope to address any update that is required during the study. It describes all the components of the data management process with each component specifying:

- Work to be performed;
- Responsible staff for the work;
- Guidelines and SOPs to be compiled with; and
- Output to be produced.

II. **Study set up:** It includes designing of case report form (CRF); CRF completion guidelines; setting up of trial data base; and validation checks.

*The designing of case report form* is crucial and the quality of data depends on quality data collection tools. They are designed during protocol development and should cover all the data specified by the protocol. The collection of extraneous data adversely affects the data quality. The following points should be kept in mind in designing CRF:

- It should be clear and concise indicating the flow of data and flow of study.
- Logically related data should be grouped together.
- Redundant data should be avoided as they invite unnecessary work for the site staff and unnecessary need for checking data consistency.
- Data based on the same measurement should be collected only once.
- Raw data is preferable. Date of birth is preferable over age.

- Data in coded form is preferable as it minimizes errors and reduces processing time.
- Coded format: multiple or single choice down list. 1 for yes, 2 for no, and 3 for not sure. This should be consistent throughout the CRF.
- It is necessary to minimize free text.

**CRF**: A CRF is designed by the CDM team. The data fields are clearly defined and consistent throughout. The type of data to be entered must be evident from CRF.

The *CRF Completion Guidelines*: The filling instructions should be made available to the site investigators for error free data acquisition. Full and accurate completion of CRF provides quality data, having fewer queries and quicker validation of data. The following general guidelines, if adopted, would lead to proper completion of CRF:

- All required fields are to be completed.
- Data recorded in CRF are logical.
- Free text entries are spelled correctly and clinically appropriate.
- Definition of items should be made available for those which are not directly measurable.
- Procedure should be in place for making correction of data.
- SOP for handling completed CRF, shipping of CRFs from the site to the data management centre and updating CRF completion guideline.

*Trial Database Set up:* All clinical trial data must be stored in a computer system. The database may be made in an excel spreadsheet or any other software. The aim of the database setup is to achieve high quality database, meet clinical and regulatory requirement, and to store data accurately. A poor database design adversely affects data entry, data cleaning, extraction and data storage.The database structure should facilitate ease and speed of data entry; prevention of errors in data creation and modification; efficient creation of data sets for analysis; and formats for data file requirements.

GCP requires that there should be a system to permit data change in such a way that the data changes are documented and that there is no deletion of entered data.

*Validation Checks:* Data validation is the process of testing the validity of data in accordance with the protocol specification. It is the crucial tool for each study database and must be created for all study endpoints. It helps to identify the discrepancy in the entered data. Discrepancy is defined as data point that fails to pass validation check. Discrepancies may occur due to to inconsistent data, missing data, range checks, and deviations from the protocol.

*Discrepancy Management:* It is also known as query resolution. This step requires reviewing discrepancy, investigating the reason and resolving them with documentary proof or declaring them as irresolvable.

**III.** **Training:** The sponsor or the company must ensure that all staff involved in the clinical research are qualified and trained to perform data management tasks. The effective training would ensure: regulatory compliance, performance effectiveness and job satisfaction of CDM staff.

The GCP specifies that each individual involved in conducting clinical trial should be qualified by education, training and experience to perform the assigned task.

The training needs to address the data entry (including handling of collected CRFs, CRF work flow and data entry module in the data management system) and discrepancy resolutions (including managing data discrepancies and discrepancy module in the data management system).

**IV.** **Data collection:** The data collection is done using the CRF which may be in the paper form (pCRF) or an electronic version (eCRF). These are then converted into database by means of in-house data entry. The paper CRF are filled by the investigators based on CRF filled guidelines. In eCRF system, the investigator or an assignee logs on to the CDM system and enters the data directly at the site. eCRF is better as there are less chances of errors and resolutions of discrepancy can happen faster.

*CRF dispatch*: The completed CRFs are to be prepared in batches and sent to data management centre. This must ensure blinding of subjects' identifying information such as name and address.

**V.** **Data processing:** This has the following activities at the data management centre:

- Data receipt: The data receipt may vary from fax transmission, regular mail, and courier delivery to web entry. The receipt of CRFs are to be documented and made available for data entry.

- CRFs tracking: All CRFs (received as well as which have direct entry) should be tracked. Missing CRFs should be specified. CRFs are tracked to detect missing pages too.

- Data review: CRFs are manually reviewed to detect data errors. A query sheet for data errors should be prepared.

- Data coding: This should be done as per the project protocol's requirement. MedDRA (Medical Dictionary for Regulatory Activities) is a tool for coding adverse events. Similarly, WHODD (World Health Organization Drug Dictionary) can be used for coding drug.

- Data entry: Data entry is a process of entering or transferring data from case report form to clinical data management system. The three basic types of data entry system are practiced:

  (a) Local data entry system – data entry is done on site;

  (b) Central data entry system – data entry is done at data management centre from the received CRFs; and

  (c) Web based data entry system – the data entry is done through web (secure link) using internet connection.

In order to make error free entry, the following data entry methods are advocated:

- Double data entry with independent verification: Two persons enter data and the third person resolves discrepancy between the two entries.

- Double data entry with blind verification: Two persons enter the data. The second person (unaware of the values entered by the first person) verifies the data and overwrite if required.

- Double data entry with interactive verification: Two persons enter data and the second person resolves discrepancy between first and second entry. The second person is aware of the value entered.

- Single data entry – review: One person enters the data and the second person reviews the entered data against the source data.

- Optical character recognition (OCR): The software is used to recognize characters from paper based CRFs or faxed images and then these data are placed directly into the database. The data obtained through OCR should be reviewed for accuracy.

Double entry method helps in getting a cleaner database compared to single data entry method. It ensures better consistency especially with paper based CRF because of lesser error rate.

- Data validation: This process is followed to detect: missing values, outliers, inconsistencies and protocol violation. Validation checks are carried out at the time of data entry and on the batches of data.

- Edit check programmes are available to identify the discrepancies in the entered data.

- Query management (Discrepancy management): This step aims to ensure rapidity of query generation and rapid resolution. The following steps are carried out: reviewing the discrepancy, investigating the reason and resolving them with documentary proof. There should be a discrepancy database.

- On the basis of discrepancy types, they are either sent to investigator for clarification or closed in-house by self-evident correction (SEC) without sending to the site. The paper based CRF and database are to be updated on resolving the issue.

- Discrepancy management is an important activity in clinical data management process.

VI. **Monitoring data quality and data safety:** The data quality should be periodically monitored as defined in the protocol. This can be achieved through site monitoring visit, training & retraining staff, and auditing.

Safety monitoring is through adverse event reporting and management of data safety monitoring board.

VII. **Audit trail:** Audit trail documents all modifications to database. These documents should be stored in open format files in a secure system.

VIII. **Data base closure (database lock):** The database closure for the study is done to ensure no manipulation of study data during final analysis. Prior to database closure, it is important to ensure: all data have been processed, quality level has been assessed, and relevant study personnel have been notified.

There should be a pre-closure check list which should be thoroughly followed as the database cannot be changed after closure.

Though in normal circumstances, data modification is not possible after database closure, there should be provision for a change with proper documentation and an audit trail and with sufficient justification.

IX. **Data storage:** Secure, efficient and accessible storage of clinical data is very important. Unauthorized access must be prevented. The collected original data like CRFs, lab data, medical notes etc., must be protected and stored in a secured place with controlled access.

There should be a system to keep the backup copies like scanning of paper documents.

X. **Security and Confidentiality:** The identifying data (name of the individual, medical record etc.) should be securely kept keeping them confidential. Copy of data cannot be distributed without investigator's consent.

XI. **Data archive:** All documents and records are to be maintained in their raw formats in a secure and stable areas (free from blood, fire protected etc.). The following documents are required to be archived:

- Original study documents
- Raw data files
- Final data files
- Audit trail
- Discrepancy management logs
- Database design specification
- Database closure documents
- Procedural variation documents

**Responsibilities of Clinical Data Management Staff:** The designations may vary from organization to organization. The common designation of the staff involved in CDM process and their responsibilities are given in the tabular form.

| Staff | Responsibilities |
|---|---|
| Data Manager | • Supervising the entire CDM process<br>• Prepares the data management plan, approves the CDM procedures, and other internal documents<br>• Controlling and allocating the database access to team members |
| Database Programmer / Designer | • Performs the CRF annotation<br>• Creates the study database<br>• Programme the edit checks for data validation<br>• Designs the data entry screens in the database and validates the edit checks with dummy data |
| Medical Coder | • Responsible for coding adverse events, medical history, co-illness, and other medications administered during the study |
| Clinical Data Coordinator | • Designs the CRF<br>• Develops CRF filling guidelines<br>• Develops the data validation plan and discrepancy management plan<br>• Develops all other CDM related documents, check lists and documents |
| Quality Control Associate | • Checks the accuracy of data entry and coordinate data audits<br>[there may be other persons authorized to conduct audit on data entered]<br>• Verifies the documentations pertaining to the procedures being followed. |
| Data Entry Associate | • Tracks the CRF pages and performs the data entry into the database |

**Principles of Good data Management Practice:** Data are critical components of a clinical research. Data quality and integrity are essential elements for a reliable data that can be used for decision making. The most effective strategy to improve the data quality is to have a data management system in place from the starting of the clinical trials. Adherence to GCP goes a long way in maintaining data quality and integrity of the trial.

The principle of ALCOA (or, ALCOA Plus) can be followed to achieve data quality. A stands for Attributable, L stands for Legible, C stands for Contemporaneous; O for Original and A for Accurate. ALCOA – Plus puts additional emphasis on the attributes of being complete, consistent, enduring and available.

- Attributable: Information is captured in the record so that it is uniquely identified having being executed. Who acquired the data or performed an action and when?
- Legible: Data are readable and understandable. This provides a clear picture of sequencing of steps or events in the record.
- Contemporaneous: Data are recorded at the time of generation or observation.
- Original: The first or source capture of data or information. Whether it is just a print out or observation or a certified copy.
- Accurate: Data are correct, truthful, complete, valid and reliable. Achieving the goal of accurate data requires adequate procedures, process, systems, and controls that comprise the quality management system.

Complete means all data are present. Consistent means that all elements of record such as the sequence of events, follow -on are dated, or time stamped in expected sequence. Enduring means data are available on proven storage media either in paper or electronic form.

*Strategies to ensure Data Integrity*: The following factors, if developed, managed or redressed, will ensure generation of high quality data in a clinical research:

- Well-designed protocol,
- Risk based monitoring plan,
- Security measures on electronic data collection documents,
- Corrective and preventive actions,
- Delegating tasks and managing personnel,
- Training personnel,
- Conducting independent internal investigations,
- Hiring Clinical Research organizations,
- Hiring third party auditors.

Good data management practices are the totality of organized measures that should be in place to collectively and individually ensure that data and records are secure, attributable, legible, traceable, permanent, contemporaneously recorded, original and accurate.

**Clinical Data Management Tools:** CDMS is a tool used to handle huge amount of data generated during clinical trials. Both commercial and open source software are used. Examples of commercial software are ORACLE CLINICAL, CLINTRIAL, MACRO, RAVE and eClinical Suite. The examples of free open source tools are Openclinica, OpenCDMS, TrialDB and PhOSCo. MS Access and MS Excel are also useful.

Data management is a critical component in a clinical research. The sponsor or PI should be responsible for keeping CDM system in place to ensure GCP compliant data.

Press Reports on Indian Companies under Scanner for Inappropriate Data Management Issues:

- Alkem Labs accused of fudging trial data by German Regulator: The Laboratories have been accused by Germany's health egulator of fudging data on clinical trials of an antibiotic and process disorder drug [Reuters, 15th April, 2016]. The company is accused of 'International misrepresentation' of data and duplicated the results of electrocardiogram (ECG) reading of patients in trials.
- European Union bans 700 generic drugs for manipulation of trials by GVK Biosciences [25th July 2015] – EMA's committee for medicinal products for human use had examined the marketing authorization given to over 1000 generic drugs from EU member nations on the basis of bioequivalence studies conducted by GVK Biosciences during period between 2004 and 2014 after an inspection of companies facilities in Hyderabad by the French Medicines Agency (ANSM) in May last year showed 'Systematic manipulation of clinical trial data' . The inspection revealed 'Data manipulation of ECGs during conduct of some studies of generic medicines.
- Selmer gets WHO notice of concern over violation of ideal laboratory and clinical practices [ET Bureau, 25th April 2016] – WHO noted "four FDA studies and one WHO study have questionable data which cannot be physiologically explained".

## Key Points to Remember

- In clinical research, data are crucial components not only for receiving regulatory approval but also to take clinical decisions in post approval period.
- Data are information or observations that are associated with a particular research project including specimens, technologies and the products.
- Data collection provides the information necessary to develop and justify research. Data collection is reliable when this is done in a consistent and comprehensive manner throughout the course of study.
- Data management is a critical component in a clinical research. The sponsor should be responsible for keeping clinical data management system in place for the study.
- CDMS is the process of collection, cleaning and management of subject data in compliance with GCP requirement.
- CDMS begins with the establishment of data management group and ends with delivery of quality database.
- Database must be accurate, secure, reliable and ready for analysis.
- Appropriate designing of case report form is a crucial component as the quality of data depends on the data collection tool. CRF is to be filled up as per the filling up guidelines developed.
- All staff involved in clinical research should be suitably qualified and trained to perform the data management task.
- Double entry method of data entry is preferable to single entry system as the former ensures better consistency and with lesser errors.
- Data manager has the responsibility of supervising the entire CDM process. Some of the other important persons involved are: database programmer, medical coder, clinical data coordinator, quality control associate and data entry associate.
- Principles of ALCOA should be followed to generate quality database.
- Many software (commercial as well as open access) are available for clinical data management.

# APPENDICES

# GLOSSARY OF TERMS

- **Accurate:** The data are correct, truthful, complete, valid and reliable.

- **Adverse Drug Reaction:** All noxious and unintended responses to a medicinal product related to any dose where a causal relationship is at least a reasonable possibility.

- **Adverse Event**: Any untoward (unfavourable and unintended) medical occurrence in a test subject administered a pharmaceutical product which does not necessarily have a causal relationship with the treatment.

- **ALCOA:** Acronym for Attributable, Legible, Contemporaneous, Original and Accurate.

- **$AUC_{0-t}$:** Area under plasma-concentration curve from 0 time to time t.

- **Audit Trail**: This is a form of metadata that contains information associated with action related to creation, modification and deletion of data record.

- **Backup:** Copy of one or more electronic files created as alternative in case original is lost or unusable.

- **Beneficence:** Ethical obligation to maximise benefit and to minimise harm.

- **Bioavailability:** The relative amount of drug from an administered dosage form which enters the systemic circulation and the rate at which the drug appears in the systemic circulation.

- **Bioequivalence:** The comparison of bioavailabilities of different formulations or drug products. Bioequivalence of a drug product is achieved if its extent and rate of absorption is not statistically significantly different from those of the reference product when administered at the same molar dose.

- **Blinding:** The procedure, in which one or more parties to the trial are kept unaware of treatment assignment(s). In single-blinding, the subjects are being unaware and in double blinding, the subject(s), investigator(s), monitor are kept unaware of treatment assignment(s).

- **Case Report Form (CRF):** A printed, optical, or electronic document designed to record all of the protocol required information to be reported to the sponsor on each trial subject.

- **Clinical Data Management System:** The process of collection, cleaning, and management of subject data in compliance with GCP requirement.

- **Clinical Research Organization (CRO):** An organization contracted by the sponsor to perform one or more of a sponsor's trial – related duties and functions.

- **Clinical Research:** The study on human beings. This includes both observational and intervention studies.

- **Clinical Trial**: A systemic study of pharmaceutical products in human subject(s), in order to discover or verify the clinical, pharmacological (including pharmacodynamic/pharmacokinetic), and/or adverse effects, with the object of determining their safety and/or efficacy.

- **$C_{max}$:** Maximum drug concentration achieved in systemic circulation following drug administration.

- **Cohort:** A group of people studied to determine the outcome after exposure to a drug.

- **Confidentiality**: The record of private information obtained would not be disclosed to others without following the appropriate procedure.

- **Data Integrity**: Degree to which data are complete, consistent, accurate, trust worthy and reliable.

- **Data Quality**: This refers to the essential characteristics of each piece of data and quality data should be ALCOA.

- **Data Safety Monitoring Board**: A body responsible for monitoring safety and efficacy data.

- **Database:** Collection of data suitably arranged for retrieval and analysis.

- **Drug Product:** A formulated drug substance ready for use.

- **Drug Regulatory Authority:** The government body that has power to regulate clinical trials or clinical research. DCGI is the authority for India.

- **Drug Substance:** A drug substance (not formulated one).

- **Effectiveness:** A measure of effect of medicine in actual use.

- **Efficacy:** The ability of medicine to bring about the intended beneficial effect on individual under ideal condition of use (clinical trial).

- **Ethics:** The rules or standard governing the conduct of individuals (principle of right conduct).

- **Good Clinical Practice:** A process that incorporates established ethical and scientific quality standards for the design, conduct, recording and reporting of clinical research involving participation of human subjects. Compliance with GCP provides public assurance that the rights, safety, and well being of research subjects are protected and respected in consistent with ethical guidelines and ensures the integrity of clinical research data.

- **Good Data Management Practice:** Totality of organised measures that should be in place to collectively and individually ensure that data and records are secure, attributable, legible, traceable, permanent, contempora- neously recorded, original and accurate.

- **Good Laboratory Practice:** This is the standard required to assure the quality and integrity of non-clinical data submitted in support of research permits or marketing application.

- **Independent Ethics Committee (IEC):** An independent body (review board, committee) constituted of medical and non-medical members whose responsibility is to ensure the protection of rights, safety and well being of human subjects involved in a clinical trial and to provide public assurance of that protection by reviewing and approving the trial protocol including provision of informed consent of the trial subjects.

- **Informed Consent:** A process by which a subject voluntarily confirms his/her willingness to participate in a particular trial, after having been informed of all aspects of the trial that are relevant to the subject's decision to participate.

- **Institutional Review Board:** An independent body constituted of medical, scientific, and non-scientific members, whose responsibility is to ensure the protection of rights, safety, and well beings of human subjects participating in clinical research and review, approve, and continue approving clinical research protocol including other documents related to clinical research.

- **International Non-Proprietary Name (INN):** Generic name of the drug substance.

- **Investigational Pharmaceutical Product:** The medicine under evaluation for safety and efficacy.

- **Investigator:** A person responsible for the conduct of clinical trial at a trial site. When more than one person is involved, the leader of the team is principal investigator.

- **Lag phase:** Delayed stage.

- **LD$_{50}$:** Dose required to kill 50% of the tested population.

- **Monitoring:** The act of overseeing the progress of a clinical trial in an attempt of ensuring that it is conducted, recorded, and reported in accordance with the protocol, Standard Operating Procedures (SOPs), Good Clinical Practice (GCP), and the applicable regulatory requirement(s).

- **New Drug:** A drug which has not been used to a significant extent and has not been recognised as safe and effective. It continues to be considered as new drug for a period of four years from its first approval or inclusion in Indian Pharmacopoeia.

- **Non-maleficence:** Do no harm.

- **Over The Counter (OTC) Medicines:** The medicines available to buy without prescription.

- **Periodic Safety Update Report (PSUR):** A periodic summary of safety information required to be submitted to the drug regulatory authority.

- **Pharmaceutical Equivalents:** Drug Products that contain the identical amounts of identical active ingredient (same salt or ester of the same therapeutic moiety), in identical dosage forms, but not necessarily containing the same active ingredients.

- **Pharmacokinetics:** The rate at which drug concentration changes in the different body fluids and tissues in the dynamic system of liberation, absorption, distribution, body storage, binding, metabolism, and excretion.

- **Pharmacovigilance:** The science and activities relating to the detection, assessment, understanding and prevention of adverse effects or any other drug related problem.

- **Placebo:** A dummy product (without pharmaceutical active substance) looking similar to the investigational pharmaceutical product.

- **Post Marketing Surveillance**: Monitoring of Adverse Drug Event after marketing approval of the drug product.

- **Privacy:** Each individual should have the right to control personal and sensitive information about him/her. Privacy implies that such information will not be disclosed without the knowledge or permission of the individual.

- **Protocol**: A document that describes the objective(s), design, methodology, statistical considerations, and organization of clinical trial.

- **Quality Assurance**: All those planned and systemic actions that are established to ensure that the trial is performed and the data are generated, documented, and reported in compliance with Good Clinical practices and applicable regulatory requirements.

- **Quality Control:** The operational techniques and activities under taken within the quality assurance system to verify that the requirements for quality of the trial related activities have been fulfilled.

- **Quality:** Quality is a measure of ability of a product, process or service to satisfy stated or implied needs.

- **Randomization**:  The process of assigning trial subjects to treatment or control groups using an element of chance to determine the assignments in order to reduce bias.

- **Regulatory Authority**: Drugs Controller General (India) (DCGI).

- **Serious Adverse Event:** Any untoward medical occurrence at any dose: that results in death, is life threatening, requires inpatient hospitalization or prolongation of existing hospitalization, results in persistent or significant disability/incapacity, or is a congenital anomaly or birth defect.

- **Signal:** Reported information on a possible causal relationship between an adverse event and a drug, the relationship being unknown or incompletely documented previously, that is recognised as worthy of further exploration and continued surveillance.

- **Sponsor:** An individual, company, institution, organization which takes responsibility for the initiation, management, and/or financing of a clinical trial.

- **Standard Operating Procedure (SOP):** Detailed, written instructions to achieve uniformity of the performance of a specific function.

- **Supra – bioavailability:** The test product displays an appreciably larger bioavailability than the reference product.

- **Sustained Release Dosage Form:** Modified release dosage forms where liberation (drug release) rate constant is smaller than the unrestricted absorption rate constant.

- **Therapeutic Equivalent**: Drug product that contains the same active substance or therapeutic moiety and, clinically show the same efficacy and safety.

- **$T_{max}$:** Time required to achieving maximum drug concentration in systemic circulation.

# APPENDICES OF SCHEDULE Y

## DATA TO BE SUBMITTED ALONG WITH THE APPLICATION TO CONDUCT CLINICALTRIALS/IMPORT/MANUFACTURE OF NEW DRUGS FOR MARKETING IN THE COUNTRY

1. **Introduction:** A brief description of the drug and the therapeutic class to which it belongs.

2. **Chemical and Pharmaceutical Information**

   2.1.  Information on active ingredients.

   Drug information (Generic Name, Chemical Name or INN)

   2.2.  Physicochemical Data

   (a)  Chemical name and Structure

   Empirical formula

   Molecular weight

   (b)  Physical properties

   Description

   Solubility

   Rotation

   Partition coefficient

   Dissociation constant

   2.3.  Analytical Data

   Elemental analysis

   Mass spectrum

   NMR spectra

   IR spectra

   UV spectra

   Polymorphic identification

   2.4.  Complete monograph specification including

   Identification Identity/quantification of impurities

   Enantiomeric purity

   Assay

2.5. Validations

Assay method

Impurity estimation method

Residual solvent/other volatile impurities (OVI) estimation method

2.6. StabilityStudies (for details refer Appendix IX)

Final release specification

Reference standard characterization

Material safety data sheet

2.7. Data on Formulation

Dosage form

Composition

Master manufacturing formula- Details of the formulation (including inactive ingredients)

In process quality control check

Finished product specification

Excipient compatibility study

Validation of the analytical method

Comparative evaluation with international brand(s) or approved Indian brands, if applicable Pack presentation

Dissolution

Assay

Impurities

Content uniformity

pH

Force degradation study

Stability evaluation in market intended pack at proposed storage conditions

Packing specifications

Process validation: When the application is for clinical trials only, the international non-proprietary name (INN) or generic name, drug category, dosage form and data supporting stability of the intended container-closure system for the duration of the clinical trial (information covered in item nos. 2.1, 2.3, 2.6, 2.7) are required.

3. **Animal Pharmacology** (for details refer Appendix IV)

   3.1. Summary

   3.2. Specific pharmacological actions

   3.3. General pharmacological actions

   3.4. Follow-up and Supplemental SafetyPharmacology Studies

   3.5. Pharmacokinetics: absorption, distribution; metabolism; excretion

4. **Animal Toxicology** (for details refer Appendix III)

   4.1. General Aspects

   4.2. Systemic Toxicity Studies

   4.3. Male Fertility Study

   4.4. Female Reproduction and Developmental Toxicity Studies

   4.5. Local toxicity

   4.6. Allergenicity/Hypersensitivity

   4.7. Genotoxicity

   4.8. Carcinogenicity

5. **Human / Clinical pharmacology** (Phase I)

   5.1. Summary

   5.2. Specific Pharmacological effects

   5.3. General Pharmacological effects

   5.4. Pharmacokinetics; absorption, distribution, metabolism, excretion

   5.5. Pharmacodynamics/early measurement of drug activity

6. **Therapeutic Exploratory Trials** (Phase II)

   6.1. Summary

   6.2. Study report(s) as given in Appendix II

7. **Therapeutic Confirmatory Trials** (Phase III)

   7.1. Summary

   7.2. Individual study reports with listing of sites and Investigators.

8. **Special Studies**

   8.1. Summary

   8.2. Bio-availability/Bio-equivalence.

8.3. Other studies e.g. geriatrics, paediatrics, pregnant or nursing women

**9. Regulatory Status in other Countries**

9.1. Countries where the drug is:
   (a) Marketed
   (b) Approved
   (c) Approved as IND
   (d) Withdrawn, if any, with reasons

9.2. Restrictions on use, if any, in countries where marketed/approved

9.3. Free sale certificate or certificate of analysis, as appropriate.

**10. Prescribing Information**

10.1. Proposed full prescribing information

10.2. Drafts of labels and cartons

**11. Samples and Testing Protocol/s**

11.1. Samples of pure drug substance and finished product (an equivalent of 50 clinical doses, or more number of clinical doses if prescribed by the Licensing Authority), with testing protocol/s, full impurity profile and release specifications.

**Notes:** 1. All items may not be applicable to all drugs. For explanation, refer text of Schedule Y.

2. For requirements of data to be submitted with application for clinical trials refer text of this Schedule.

# APPENDIX - IA

**DATA REQUIRED TO BE SUBMITTED BY AN APPLICANT FOR GRANT OF PERMISSION TO IMPORT AND/OR MANUFACTURE A NEW DRUG ALREADY APPROVED IN THE COUNTRY**

1. **Introduction**

   A brief description of the drug and the therapeutic class

2. **Chemical and Pharmaceutical Information**

   2.1 Chemical name, code name or number, if any; non-proprietary or generic name, if any, structure; physico-chemical properties

   2.2 Dosage form and its composition

   2.3 Test specifications

   (a) active ingredients

   (b) inactive ingredients

   2.4 Tests for identification of the active ingredients and method of its assay

   2.5 Outline of the method of manufacture of active ingredients

   2.6 Stability data

3. **Marketing Information**

   3.1 Proposed package insert / promotional literature

   3.2 Draft specimen of the label and carton

4. **Special Studies Conducted with Approval of Licensing Authority**

   4.1 Bioavailability / Bioequivalence and comparative dissolution studies for oral dosage forms

   4.2 Sub-acute animal toxicity studies for intravenous infusions and injectables

## STRUCTURE, CONTENTS AND FORMAT FOR CLINICAL STUDY REPORTS

1. **Title Page:** This page should contain information about the title of the study, the protocol code, name of the investigational product tested, development phase, indication studied, a brief description of the trial design, the start and end date of patient accrual and the names of the Sponsor and the participating Institutes (Investigators).

2. **Study Synopsis (1 to 2 pages):** A brief overview of the study from the protocol development to the trial closure should be given here. This section will only summarize the important conclusions derived from the study.

3. **Statement of compliance with the 'Guidelines for Clinical Trials on Pharmaceutical Products in India:** GCP Guidelines' issued by the Central Drugs Standard Control Organization, Ministry of Health, Government of India.

4. **List of Abbreviations and Definitions**

5. **Table of Contents**

6. **Ethics Committee:** [The Drugs and Cosmetics Act, 1940 and Rules, 1945 Sch. Y]: This section should document that the study was conducted in accordance with the ethical principles of Declaration of Helsinki. A detailed description of the Ethics Committee constitution and date(s) of approvals of trial documents for each of the participating sites should be provided. A declaration should state that EC notifications as per Good Clinical Practice Guidelines issued by Central Drugs Standard Control Organization and Ethical Guidelines for Biomedical Research on Human Subjects, issued by Indian Council of Medical Research have been followed.

7. **Study Team:** Briefly describe the administrative structure of the study (Investigators, site staff, Sponsor/ designates, Central laboratory etc.).

8. **Introduction:** A brief description of the product development rationale should be given here.

9. **Study Objective:** A statement describing the overall purpose of the study and the primary and secondary objectives to be achieved should be mentioned here.

10. **Investigational Plan:** This section should describe the overall trial design, the Subject selection criteria, the treatment procedures, blinding / randomization techniques if any, allowed/ disallowed concomitant treatment, the efficacy and safety criteria assessed, the data quality assurance procedures and the statistical methods planned for the analysis of the data obtained.

11. **Trial Subjects:** A clear accounting of all trial Subjects who entered the study will be given here. Mention should also be made of all cases that were dropouts or protocol deviations. Enumerate the patients screened, randomised, and prematurely discontinued. State reasons for premature discontinuation of therapy in each applicable case.

12. **Efficacy Evaluation:** The results of evaluation of all the efficacy variables will be described in this section with appropriate tabular and graphical representation. A brief description of the demographic characteristics of the trial patients should also be provided along with a listing of patients and observations excluded from efficacy analysis.

13. **Safety Evaluation:** This section should include the complete list of:

    13.1  All serious adverse events, whether expected or unexpected and

    13.2  Unexpected advese events whether serious or not (compiled from data received as per Appendix XI). The comparison of adverse events across study groups may be presented in a tabular or graphical form. This section should also give a brief narrative of all important events considered related to the investigational product.

14. **Discussion and overall Conclusion:** Discussion of the important conclusions derived from the trial and scope for further development.

15. **List of References:**

16. **Appendices:** List of Appendices to the Clinical Trial Report

    (a)  Protocol and amendments

(b) Specimen of Case Record Form

(c) Investigators' name(s) with contact addresses, phone, e-mail etc.

(d) Patient data listings

(e) List of trial participants treated with the investigational product

(f) Discontinued participants

(g) Protocol deviations

(h) CRFs of cases involving death and life threatening adverse event cases

(i) Publications from the trial

(j) Important publications referenced in the study

(k) Audit certificate, if available

(l) Investigator's certificate that he/she has read the report and that the report accurately describes the conduct and the results of the study.

## ANIMAL TOXICOLOGY (NON-CLINICAL TOXICITY STUDIES)

1. **General Principles:** Toxicity studies should comply with the norms of Good Laboratory Practice (GLP). Briefly, these studies should be performed by suitably trained and qualified staff employing properly calibrated and standardized equipment of adequate size and capacity. Studies should be done as per written protocols with modifications (if any) verifiable retrospectively. Standard operating procedures (SOPs) should be followed for all managerial and laboratory tasks related to these studies. Test substances and test systems (*in-vitro or in-vivo*) should be properly characterized and standardized. All documents belonging to each study, including its approved protocol, raw data, draft report, final report, and histology slides and paraffin tissue blocks should be preserved for a minimum of 5 years after marketing of the drug. Toxicokinetic studies (generation of pharmacokinetic data either as an integral component of the conduct of non-clinical toxicity studies or in specially designed studies) should be conducted to assess the systemic exposure achieved in animals and its relationship to dose level and the time course of the toxicity study. Other objectives of toxicokinetic studies include obtaining data to relate the exposure achieved in toxicity studies to toxicological findings and contribute to the assessment of the relevance of these findings to clinical safety, to support the choice of species and treatment regimen in nonclinical toxicity studies and to provide information which, in conjunction with the toxicity findings, contributes to the design of subsequent non-clinical toxicity studies.

   **1.1    Systemic Toxicity Studies**

   **1.1.1    Single-dose Toxicity Studies:** These studies (see Appendix I item 4.2) should be carried out in 2 rodent species (mice and rats) using the same route as intended for humans. In addition, unless the intended route of administration in humans is only intravenous, at least one more route should be used in one of the species to ensure systemic absorption of the drug. This route should depend on the nature of the drug. A limit of 2g/kg (or 10 times the normal dose that is intended in humans, whichever is higher) is recommended for oral dosing. Animals should be observed for 14 days after the drug administration, and minimum lethal dose (MLD) and maximum tolerated dose (MTD) should be established. If possible, the target organ of toxicity should also be determined. Mortality should be observed for up to 7 days after parenteral administration and up to 14 days after oral administration. Symptoms, signs and mode of death should be reported, with appropriate macroscopic and microscopic findings where necessary. $LD_{10}$ and $LD_{50}$ should be reported preferably with 95 percent confidence limits. If $LD_{50}$s cannot be determined, reasons for the same should be stated.

The dose causing severe toxic manifestations or death should be defined in the case of cytotoxic anticancer agents, and the post-dosing observation period should be up to 14 days. Mice should first be used for determination of MTD. Findings should then be confirmed in rat for establishing linear relationship between toxicity and body surface area. In case of nonlinearity, data of the more sensitive species should be used to determine the Phase I starting dose. Where rodents are known to be poor predictors of human toxicity (e.g., antifolates), or where the cytotoxic drug acts by a novel mechanism of action, MTD should be established in non-rodent species.

**1.1.2 Repeated-dose Systemic Toxicity Studies**: These studies (see Appendix I, item 4.2) should be carried out in at least two mammalian species, of which one should be a non- rodent. Dose ranging studies should precede the 14-, 28-, 90- or 180- day toxicity studies. Duration of the final systematic toxicity study will depend on the duration, therapeutic indication and scale of the proposed clinical trial (see item 1.8). If a species is known to metabolize the drug in the same way as humans, it should be preferred for toxicity studies.

In repeated-dose toxicity studies the drug should be administered 7 days a week by the route intended for clinical use. The number of animals required for these studies, i.e. the minimum number of animals on which data should be available, is shown in Item 1.9.

Wherever applicable, a control group of animals given the vehicle alone should be included, and three other groups should be given graded doses of the drug. The highest dose should produce observable toxicity; the lowest dose should not cause observable toxicity, but should be comparable to the intended therapeutic dose in humans or a multiple of it. To make allowance for the sensitivity of the species the intermediate dose should cause some symptoms, but not gross toxicity or death, and should be placed logarithmically between the other two doses.

The parameters to be monitored and recorded in long-term toxicity studies should include behavioural, physiological, biochemical and microscopic observations. In case of parenteral drug administration, the sites of injection should be subjected to gross and microscopic examination. Initial and final electrocardiogram and fundus examination should be carried out in the non-rodent species.

In the case of cytotoxic anticancer agents dosing and study design should be in accordance with the proposed clinical schedule in terms of days of exposure and number of cycles. Two rodent species may be tested for initiating Phase I trials. A non-rodent species should be added if the drug has a novel mechanism of action, or if permission for Phase II, III or marketing is being sought.

For most compounds, it is expected that single dose-tissue distribution studies with sufficient sensitivity and specificity will provide an adequate assessment of tissue distribution and the potential for accumulation. Thus, repeated dose tissue distribution studies should not be required uniformly for all compounds and should only be conducted when appropriate data cannot be derived from other sources. Repeated dose studies may be appropriate under certain circumstances based on the data from single dose tissue distribution studies, toxicity and toxico kinetic studies. The studies may be most appropriate for compounds which have an apparently long half-life, incomplete elimination or unanticipated organ toxicity.

**Notes:**

**(i) Single Dose Toxicity Study:** Each group should contain at least 5 animals of either sex. At least four graded doses should be given. Animals should be exposed to the test substance in a single bolus or by continuous infusion or several doses within 24 hours. Animals should be observed for 14 days. Signs of intoxication, effect on body weight, gross pathological changes should be reported. It is desirable to include histo-pathology of grossly affected organs, if any.

**(ii) Dose-ranging Study:** Objectives of this study include the identification of target organ of toxicity and establishment of MTD for subsequent studies.

(a) *Rodents*: Study should be performed in one rodent species (preferably rat) by the proposed clinical route of administration. At least four graded doses including control should be given, and each dose group as well as the vehicle control should consist of a minimum of 5 animals of each sex. Animals should be exposed to the test substance daily for 10 consecutive days. Highest dose should be the maximum tolerated dose of single-dose study. Animals should be observed daily for signs of intoxication (general appearance, activity and behaviour etc), and periodically for the body weight and laboratory parameters. Gross examination of viscera and microscopic examination of affected organs should be done.

(b) *Non-rodents*: One male and one female are to be taken for ascending Phase MTD study. Dosing should start after initial recording of cage-side and laboratory. Single-dose Toxicity Studies: These studies (see Appendix I item 4.2) should be carried or MTD (whichever is less), and dose escalation in suitable steps should be done every third day after drawing the samples for laboratory parameters. Dose should be lowered appropriately when clinical or laboratory evidence of toxicity are observed. Administration of test substance should then continue for 10 days at the well-tolerated dose level following which, samples for laboratory parameters should be taken. Sacrifice, autopsy and microscopic examination of affected tissues should be performed as in the case of rodents.

(iii) **14-28 Day Repeated-dose Toxicity Studies:** One rodent (6-10/sex/group) and one non-rodent (2-3/sex/group) species are needed. Daily dosing by proposed clinical route at three dose levels should be done with highest dose having observable toxicity, mid-dose between high and low dose, and low dose. The doses should preferably be multiples of the effective dose and free from toxicity. Observation parameters should include cage- side observations, body weight changes, food/water intake, blood biochemistry, haematology, and gross and microscopic studies of all viscera and tissues.

(iv) **90-Day Repeated-dose Toxicity Studies**: One rodent (15-30/sex/group) and one non-rodent (4-6/sex/group) species are needed. Daily dosing by proposed clinical route at three graded dose levels should be done. In addition to the control a "high-dose reversal" group and its control group should be also included. Parameters should include signs of intoxication (general appearance, activity and behaviour etc), body weight, food intake, blood biochemical parameters, haematological values, urine analysis, organ weights, gross and microscopic study of viscera and tissues. Half the animals in "reversal" groups (treated and control) should be sacrificed after 14 days of stopping the treatment. The remaining animals should be sacrificed after 28 days of stopping the treatment or after the recovery of signs and/or clinical pathological changes – whichever comes later, and evaluated for the parameters used for the main study.

(v) **180-Day Repeated-dose Toxicity Studies**: One rodent (15-30/sex/group) and one non-rodent (4-6/sex/group) species are needed. At least 4 groups, including control, should be taken. Daily dosing by proposed clinical route at three graded dose levels should be done. Parameters should include signs of intoxication, body weight, food intake, blood biochemistry, hematology, urine analysis, organ weights, gross and microscopic examination of organs and tissues.

**1.2 Male Fertility Study:** One rodent species (preferably rat) should be used. Dose selection should be done from the results of the previous 14 or 28-day toxicity study in rat. Three dose groups, the highest one showing minimal toxicity in systemic studies, and a control group should be taken. Each group should consist of 6 adult male animals. Animals should be treated with the test substance by the intended route of clinical use for minimum 28 days and maximum 70 days before they are paired with female animals of proven fertility in a ratio of 1:2 for mating.

Drug treatment of the male animals should continue during pairing. Pairing should be continued till the detection of vaginal plug or 10 days, whichever is earlier. Females getting thus pregnant should be examined for their fertility index after 13 days of gestation. All the male animals should be sacrificed at the end of the study. Weights of each testis and epididymis should be separately recorded. Sperms from one epididymis should be examined for their motility and morphology. The other epididymis and both testis should be examined for their histology.

**1.3** **Female Reproduction and Developmental Toxicity Studies**: These studies (see Appendix I, item 4.4) need to be carried out for all drugs proposed to be studied or used in women of child bearing age. Segment I, II and III studies (see below) are to be performed in albino mice or rats, and segment II study should include albino rabbits also, as a second test species.

On the occasion, when the test article is not compatible with the rabbit (e.g. antibiotics which are effective against gram positive, anaerobic organisms and protozoas) the Segment II data in the mouse may be substituted.

**1.3.1** **Female Fertility Study (Segment I)**: The study should be done in one rodent species (rat preferred). The drug should be administered to both males and females, beginning from a sufficient number of days (28 days in males and 14 days in females) before mating. Drug treatment should continue during mating and, subsequently, during the gestation period. Three graded doses should be used, the highest dose (usually the MTD obtained from previous systemic toxicity studies) should not affect general health of the parent animals. At least 15 males and 15 females should be used per dose group. Control and the treated groups should be of similar size. The route of administration should be the same as that intended for therapeutic use.

Dams should be allowed to litter and their medication should be continued till the weaning of pups. Observations on body weight, food intake, clinical signs of intoxication, mating behaviour, progress of gestation/ parturition periods, length of gestation, parturition, postpartum health and gross pathology (and histopathology of affected organs) of dams should be recorded. The pups from both treated and control groups should be observed for general signs of intoxication, sex-wise distribution in different treatment groups, body weight, growth parameters, survival, gross examination, and autopsy. Histopathology of affected organs should be done.

**1.3.2  Teratogenicity Study (Segment II):** One rodent (preferably rat) and one non-rodent (rabbit) species are to be used. The drug should be administered throughout the period of organogenesis, using three dose levels as described for segment I. The highest dose should cause minimum maternal toxicity and the lowest one should be proportional to the proposed dose for clinical use in humans or a multiple of it. The route of administration should be the same as that intended for human therapeutic use.

The control and the treated groups should consist of at least 20 pregnant rats (or mice) and 12 rabbits, on each dose level. All foetuses should be subjected to gross examination, one of the foetuses should be examined for skeletal abnormalities and the other half for visceral abnormalities. Observation parameters should include: (Dams) signs of intoxication, effect on body weight, effect on food intake, examination of uterus, ovaries and uterine contents, number of corpora lutea, implantation sites, resorptions (if any); and for the foetuses, the total number, gender, body length, weight and gross/ visceral/ skeletal abnormalities, if any.

**1.3.3  Perinatal Study (Segment III):** This study is specially recommended if the drug is to be given to pregnant or nursing mothers for long periods or where there are indications of possible adverse effects on foetal development. One rodent species (preferably rat) is needed. Dosing at levels comparable to multiples of human dose should be done by the intended clinical route. At least 4 groups (including control), each consisting of 15 dams should be used. The drug should be administered throughout the last trimester of pregnancy (from day 15 of gestation) and then the dose that causes low foetal loss should be continued throughout lactation and weaning. Dams should then be sacrificed and examined as described below.

One male and one female from each litter of F1 generation (total 15 males and 15 females in each group) should be selected at weaning and treated with vehicle or test substance (at the dose levels described above) throughout their periods of growth to sexual maturity, pairing, gestation, parturition and lactation. Mating performance and fertility of F1 generation should thus be evaluated to obtain the F2 generation whose growth parameters should be monitored till weaning.

Animals should be sacrificed at the end of the study and the observation parameters should include (Dams) body weight, food intake, general signs of intoxication, progress of gestation/ parturition periods and gross pathology (if any); and for pups, the clinical signs, sexwise distribution in dose groups, body weight, growth parameters, gross examination, survival and autopsy (if needed) and where necessary, histopathology.

**1.4 Local Toxicity**: These studies (see Appendix I, item 4.5) are required when the new drug is proposed to be used by some special route (other than oral) in humans. The drug should be applied to an appropriate site (e.g., skin or vaginal mucous membrane) to determine local effects in a suitable species. Typical study designs for these studies should include three dose levels and untreated and/ or vehicle control, preferably use of 2 species, and increasing group size with increase in duration of treatment. Where dosing is restricted due to anatomical or humane reasons, or the drug concentration cannot be increased beyond a certain level due to the problems of solubility, pH or tonicity, a clear statement to this effect should be given. If the drug is absorbed from the site of application, appropriate systemic toxicity studies will also be required.

**Notes:**

(i) **Dermal Toxicity Study**: The study should be done in rabbit and rat. Daily topical (dermal) application of test substance in its clinical dosage form should be done. Test material should be applied on shaved skin covering not less than 10% of the total body surface area. Porous gauze dressing should be used to hold liquid material in place. Formulations with different concentrations (atleast 3) of test substance, several fold higher than the clinical dosage form should be used. Period of application may vary from 7 to 90 days depending on the clinical duration of use. Where skin irritation is grossly visible in the initial studies, a recovery group should be included in the subsequent repeated-dose study. Local signs (erythema, oedema and eschar formation) as well as histological examination of sites of application should be used for evaluation of results.

(ii) **Photo-allergy or Dermal Photo-toxicity**: It should be tested by Armstrong/ Harber Test in guinea pig. This test should be done if the drug or a metabolite is related to an agent causing photosensitivity or the nature of action suggests such a potential (e.g., drugs to be used in the treatment of leucoderma). Pre-test in 8 animals should screen 4 concentrations (patch application for 2 hours ±15 min.) with and without UV exposure (10 J/cm2). Observations recorded at 24 and 48 hours should be used to ascertain highest non-irritant dose. Main test should be performed with 10 test animals and 5 controls. Induction with the dose selected from pre-test should use 0.3 ml/patch for 2 hour ±15 min. followed by 10 $J/cm^2$ of UV exposure. This should be repeated on day 0, 2,4,7,9 and 11 of the test. Animals should be challenged with the same concentration of test substance between day 20 to 24 of the test with a similar 2-hour application followed by exposure to 10 $J/cm^2$ of UV light. Examination and grading of erythema and oedema formation at the challenge sites should be done 24 and 48 hours after the challenge. A positive control like musk ambrett or psoralin should be used.

(iii) **Vaginal Toxicity Test**: Study is to be done in rabbits or dogs. Test substance should be applied topically (vaginal mucosa) in the form of pessary, cream or ointment. Six to ten animals per dose group should be taken. Higher concentrations or several daily applications of test substance should be done to achieve multiples of daily human dose. The minimum duration of drug treatment is 7 days (more according to clinical use), subject to a maximum of 30 days. Observation parameters should include swelling, closure of introitus and histopathology of vaginal wall.

(iv) **Rectal Tolerance Test**: For all preparations meant for rectal administration this test may be performed in rabbits or dogs. Six to ten animals per dose group should be taken. Formulation in volume comparable to human dose (or the maximum possible volume) should be applied once or several times daily, per rectally, to achieve administration of multiples of daily human dose. The minimum duration of application is 7 days, lowest one should be proportional to the proposed dose for clinical use in humans or a multiple may be smaller, but the drug content should be several fold higher than the proposed human dose. Observation parameters should include clinical signs (sliding on backside), signs of pain, blood and/or mucus in faeces, condition of anal region/sphincter, gross and (if required) histological examination of rectal mucosa.

(v) **Parenteral Drugs**: For products meant for intravenous or intramuscular or subcutaneous or intradermal injection the sites of injection in systemic toxicity studies should be specially examined grossly and microscopically. If needed, reversibility of adverse effects may be determined on a case to case basis.

(vi) **Ocular Toxicity Studies (for products meant for ocular instillation)**: These studies should be carried out in two species, one of which should be the albino rabbit which has a sufficiently large conjunctival sac. Direct delivery of drug onto the cornea in case of animals having small conjunctival sacs should be ensured. Liquids, ointments, gels or soft contact lenses (saturated with drug) should be used. Initial single dose application should be done to decide the exposure concentrations for repeated-dose studies and the need to include a recovery group. Duration of the final study will depend on the proposed length of human exposure subject to a maximum of 90 days. At least two different concentrations exceeding the human dose should be used for demonstrating the margin of safety. In acute studies, one eye should be used for drug administration and the other kept as control. A separate control group should be included in repeated-dose studies. Slit-lamp examination should be done to detect the changes in cornea, iris and aqueous humor. Fluorescent dyes (sodium fluorescein, 0.25 to 1.0%) should be used for detecting the defects in surface epithelium of cornea and conjunctiva. Changes in intraocular tension should be monitored by a tonometer. Histological examination of eyes should be done at the end of the study after fixation in Davidson's or Zenker's fluid.

(vii) **Inhalation Toxicity Studies**: The studies are to be undertaken in one rodent and one non-rodent species using the formulation that is to be eventually proposed to be marketed. Acute, subacute and chronic toxicity studies should be performed according to the intended duration of human exposure. Standard systemic toxicity study designs (described above) should be used. Gases and vapours should be given in whole body exposure chambers; aerosols are to be given by nose-only method. Exposure time and concentrations of test substance (limit dose of 5mg/l) should be adjusted to ensure exposure at levels comparable to multiples of intended human exposure. Three dose groups and a control (plus vehicle control, if needed) are required. Duration of exposure may vary subject to a maximum of 6 hours per day and five days a week. Food and water should be withdrawn during the period of exposure to test substance. Temperature, humidity and flow rate of exposure chamber should be recorded and reported. Evidence of exposure with test substance of particle size of 4 micron (especially for aerosols) with not less than 25% being 1 micron should be provided. Effects on respiratory rate, findings of bronchial lavage fluid examination, histological examination of respiratory passages and lung tissue should be included along with the regular parameters of systemic toxicity studies or assessment of margin of safety.

**1.5** **Allergenicity/ Hypersensitivity**: Standard tests include guinea pig maximization test (GPMT) and local lymph node assay (LLNA) in mouse. Any one of the two may be done.

**Notes:**

(i) **Guinea Pig Maximization Test**: The test is to be performed in two steps; first, determination of maximum non-irritant and minimum irritant doses, and second, the main test. The initial study will also have two components. To determine the intradermal induction dose, 4 dose levels should be tested by the same route in a batch of 4 male and 4 female animals (2 of each sex should be given Freund's adjuvant). The minimum irritant dose should be used for induction. Similarly, a topical minimum irritant dose should be determined for challenge. This should be established in 2 males and 2 females. A minimum of 6 male and 6 female animals per group should be used in the main study. One test and one control group should be used. It is preferable to have one more positive control group. Intradermal induction (day 1) coupled with topical challenge (day 21) should be done. If there is no response, re-challenge should be done 7-30 days after the primary challenge. Erythema and oedema (individual animal scores as well as maximization grading) should be used as evaluation criteria.

(ii) **Local Lymph Node Assay**: Mice used in this test should be of the same sex, either only males or only females. Drug treatment is to be given on ear skin. Three graded doses, the highest being maximum non-irritant dose plus vehicle control should be used. A minimum of 6 mice per group should be used. Test material should be applied on ear skin on three consecutive days and on day 5, the draining auricular lymph nodes should be dissected out 5 hours after i.v. H-thymidine or bromo-deoxy-uridine (BrdU). Increase in H-thymidine or BrdU incorporation should be used as the criterion for evaluation of results.

**1.6    Genotoxicity:** Genotoxic compounds, in the absence of other data, shall be presumed to be trans- species carcinogens, implying a hazard to humans. Such compounds need not be subjected to long-term carcinogenicity studies. However, if such a drug is intended to be administered for chronic illnesses or otherwise over a long period of time - a chronic toxicity study (up to one year) may be necessary to detect early tumorigenic effects.

Genotoxicity tests are *in vitro* and *in vivo* tests conducted to detect compounds which induce genetic damage directly or indirectly. These tests should enable a hazard identification with respect to damage to DNA and its fixation.

The following standard test battery is generally expected to be conducted:

(i) A test for gene mutation in bacteria.
(ii) An *in vitro* test with cytogenetic evaluation of chromosomal damage with mammalian cells or an *in vitro* mouse lymphomatic assay.
(iii) An *in vivo* test for chromosomal damage using rodent haematopoietic cells.

Other genotoxicity tests e.g. tests for measurement of DNA adducts, DNA strand breaks, DNA repair or recombination serve as options in addition to the standard battery for further investigation of genotoxicity test results obtained in the standard battery. Only under extreme conditions when one or more tests comprising the standard battery cannot be employed for technical reasons, alternative validated tests can serve as substitutes provided, sufficient scientific justification should be provided to support the argument that a given standard battery test is not appropriate.

Both *in-vitro* and *in-vivo* studies should be done. *In-vitro* studies should include Ames' Salmonella assay and chromosomal aberrations (CA) in cultured cells. *In-vivo* studies should include micronucleus assay (MNA) or CA in rodent bone marrow. Data analysis of CA should include analysis of 'gaps.'

Cytotoxic anticancer agents: Genotoxicity data are not required before Phase I and II trials. But these studies should be completed before applying for Phase III trials.

**Notes:** Ames'Test (Reverse mutation assay in Salmonella): S. typhimurium tester strains such as TA98, TA100, TA102, TA1535, TA97 or Escherichia coli WP2 uvrA or Escherichia coli WP2 uvrA (pKM101) should be used.

(i) *In-vitro* **Exposure (with and without metabolic activation, S9 mix)** should be done at a minimum of 5 log dose levels. "Solvent" and "positive" control should be used. Positive control may include 9-amino-acridine, 2-nitrofluorine, sodium azide and mitomycin C, respectively, in the tester strains mentioned above. Each set should consist of at least three replicates. A 2.5 fold (or more) increase in number of revertants in comparison to spontaneous revertants would be considered positive.

(ii) *In-vitro* **Cytogenetic Assay:** The desired level of toxicity for *in vitro* cytogenetic tests using cell lines should be greater than 50% reduction in cell number or culture confluency. For lymphocyte cultures, an inhibition of mitotic index by greater than 50% is considered sufficient. It should be performed in CHO cells or on human lymphocyte in culture. *Invitro* exposure (with and without metabolic activation, S9 mix) should be done using a minimum of 3 log doses. "Solvent" and "positive" control should be included. A positive control like Cyclophosphamide with metabolic activation and Mitomycin C for without metabolic activation should be used to give a reproducible and detectable increase in clastogenic effect over the background which demonstrates the sensitivity of the test system. Each set should consist of at least three replicates. Increased number of aberrations in metaphase chromosomes should be used as the criteria for evaluation.

(iii) *In-vivo* **Micronucleus Assay:** One rodent species (preferably mouse) is needed. Route of administration of test substance should be the same as intended for humans. Five animals per sex per dose groups should be used. At least three dose levels, plus "solvent" and "positive" control should be tested. A positive control like mitomycin C or cyclophosphamide should be used. Dosing should be done on day 1 and 2 of study followed by sacrifice of animals 6 hours after the last injection. Bone marrow from both the femora should be taken out, flushed with fetal bovine serum (20 min.), pelletted and smeared on glass slides. May Giemsa Gruenwald staining should be done and increased number of micronuclei in polychromatic erythrocytes (minimum 1000) should be used as the evaluation criteria.

(iv) *In-vivo* **Cytogenetic Assay**: One rodent species (preferably rat) is to be used. Route of administration of test substance should be the same as intended for humans. Five animals/sex/dose groups should be used. At least three dose levels, plus "solvent" and "positive" control should be tested. Positive control may include cyclophosphamide. Dosing should be done on day 1 followed by intra-peritoneal colchicine administration at 22 hours. Animals should be sacrificed 2 hours after colchicine administration. Bone marrow from both the femora should be taken out, flushed with hypotonic saline (20 min.), pelletted and resuspended in Carnoy's fluid. Once again the cells should be pelletted and dropped on clean glass slides with a Pasteur pipette. Giemsa staining should be done and increased number of aberrations in metaphase chromosomes (minimum 100) should be used as the evaluation criteria.

**1.7** **Carcinogenicity (see Appendix I, item 4.8)**: Carcinogenicity studies should be performed for all drugs that are expected to be clinically used for more than 6 months as well as for drugs used frequently in an intermittent manner in the treatment of chronic or recurrent conditions. Carcinogenicity studies are also to be performed for drugs if there is concern about their carcinogenic potential emanating from previous demonstration of carcinogenic potential in the product class that is considered relevant to humans or where structure-activity relationship suggests carcinogenic risk or when there is evidence of pre-neoplastic lesions in repeated dose toxicity studies or when long-term tissue retention of parent compound or metabolite(s) results in local tissue reactions or other pathophysiological responses. For pharmaceuticals developed to treat certain serious diseases, Licensing Authority may allow carcinogenicity testing to be conducted after marketing permission has been granted.

In instances where the life-expectancy in the indicated population is short (i.e., less than 2-3 years)- no long-term carcinogenicity studies may be required. In cases where the therapeutic agent for cancer is generally successful and life is significantly prolonged there may be later concerns regarding secondary cancers. When such drugs are intended for adjuvant therapy in tumour free patients or for prolonged use in non-cancer indications, carcinogenicity studies may be / are needed. Completed rodent carcinogenicity studies are not needed in advance of the conduct of large scale clinical trials, unless there is special concern for the patient population.

Carcinogenicity studies should be done in a rodent species (preferably rat). Mouse may be employed only with proper scientific justification. The selected strain of animals should not have a very high or very low incidence of spontaneous tumors.

Atleast three dose levels should be used. The highest dose should be sub-lethal, and it should not reduce the life span of animals by more than 10% of expected normal. The lowest dose should be comparable to the intended human therapeutic dose or a multiple of it, e.g. 2.5x; to make allowance for the sensitivity of the species. The intermediate dose should be placed logarithmically between the other two doses. An untreated control and (if indicated) a vehicle control group should be included. The drug should be administered 7 days a week for a fraction of the life span comparable to the fraction of human life span over which the drug is likely to be used therapeutically. Generally, the period of dosing should be 24 months for rats and 18 months for mice.

Observations should include macroscopic changes observed at autopsy and detailed histopathology of organs and tissues. Additional tests for carcinogenicity (short term bioassays, neonatal mouse assay or tests employing transgenic animals) may also be done depending on their applicability on a case to case basis.

**Note:** Each dose group and concurrent control group not intended to be sacrificed early should contain atleast 50 animals of each sex. A high dose sattelite group for evaluation of pathology other than neoplasia should contain 20 animals of each sex while the sattelite control group should contain 10 animals of each sex. Observation parameters should include signs of intoxication, effect on body weight, food intake, clinical chemistry parameters, hematology parameters, urine analysis, organ weights, gross pathology and detailed histopathology. Comprehensive descriptions of benign and malignant tumour development, time of their detection, site, dimensions, histological typing etc. should be given.

## 1.8 Animal toxicity requirements for clinical trials and marketing of a new drug.

| Systemic Toxicity Studies | | | |
|---|---|---|---|
| Route of administration | Duration of proposed human administration | Human Phase(s) for which study is proposed to be conducted | Long term toxicity requirements |
| Oral or Parenteral or Transdermal | Single dose or several doses in one day, Upto 1wk | I,II,III | 2sp;2wk |
| | > 1 wk but upto 2wk | I,II,III | 2sp;4wk |
| | > 2 wk but upto 4wk | I,II,III | 2sp;12wk |
| | Over 1mo | I,II,III | 2sp;24wk |
| Inhalation (general anaesthetics, aerosols) | Upto 2 wk | I,II,III | 2sp;1mo; (Exposure time 3h/d, 5d/wk) |
| | Upto 4wk | I,II,III | 2sp;12wk, (Exposure time 6h/d, 5d/wk) |
| | > 4wk | I,II,III | 2sp;24wk, (Exposure time 6h/d, 5d/wk) |
| **Local Toxicity Studies** | | | |
| Dermal | Upto 2 wk | I,II | 1sp;4wk |
| | | III | 2sp;4wk |
| | > 24 wk | I,II,III | 2sp;12wk |
| **Systemic Toxicity Studies** | | | |
| Ocular or Otic or Nasal | Upto 2 wk | I,II | 1sp;4wk |
| | | III | 2sp;4wk |
| | > 2 wk | I,II,III | 2sp;12wk |
| Vaginal or Rectal | Upto 2 wk | I,II | 1sp;4wk |
| | | III | 2sp;4wk |
| | > 2 wk | I,II,III | 2sp;12wk |

| **Special Toxicity Studies** |
|---|
| Male Fertility Study:<br>☐ Phase I, II, III in male volunteers/patients |
| Female Reproduction and Developmental Toxicity Studies:<br>☐ Segment II studies in 2 species; Phase II, III involving female patients of child-bearing age.<br>☐ Segment I study; Phase III involving female patients of child-bearing age.<br>☐ Segment III study; Phase III for drugs to be given to pregnant or nursing mothers for long periods or where there are indications of possible adverse effects on foetal development. |
| Allergenicity/Hypersensitivity:<br>☐ Phase I, II, III - when there is a cause of concern or for parenteral drugs (including dermal application) |
| Photo-allergy or dermal photo-toxicity:<br>☐ Phase I, II, III - if the drug or a metabolite is related to an agent causing photosensitivity or the nature of action suggests such a potential. |
| Genotoxicity:<br>☐ *In-vitro* studies - Phase I<br>☐ Both *in-vitro* and *in-vivo* - Phase II, III |
| Carcinogenicity:<br>☐ Phase III - when there is a cause for concern, or when the drug is to be used for more than 6 months. |

**Abbreviations:** sp-species; mo-month; wk-week; d-day; h-hour; I, II, III - Phases of clinical trial;

**Note**:

1. Animal toxicity data generated in other countries may be accepted and may not be asked to be repeated / duplicated in India on a case to case basis depending upon the quality of data and the credentials of the laboratory (ies) where such data has been generated.

2. Requirements for fixed dose combinations are given in Appendix VI.

## 1.9 Number of animals required for repeated-dose toxicity studies

| Group | 14-28 days | | | | 84-182 days | | | |
|---|---|---|---|---|---|---|---|---|
| | Rodent (Rat) | | Non-rodent (Dog or Monkey) | | Rodent (Rat) | | Non-rodent (Dog or Monkey) | |
| | M | F | M | F | M | F | M | F |
| Control | 6-10 | 6-10 | 2-3 | 2-3 | 15-30 | 15-30 | 4-6 | 4-6 |
| Low dose | 6-10 | 6-10 | 2-3 | 2-3 | 15-30 | 15-30 | 4-6 | 4-6 |
| Intermediate dose | 6-10 | 6-10 | 2-3 | 2-3 | 15-30 | 15-30 | 4-6 | 4-6 |
| High dose | 6-10 | 6-10 | 2-3 | 2-3 | 15-30 | 15-30 | 4-6 | 4-6 |

## 1.10 Laboratory parameters to be included in toxicity studies.

| Haematological parameters | | | |
|---|---|---|---|
| • Haemoglobin | • Total RBC Count | • Haematocrit | • Reticulocyte Count |
| • Total WBC Count | • Differential WBC Count | • Platelet Count | • Terminal Bone Marrow Examination |
| • ESR (Non-rodents only) | • General Blood Picture:  A special mention of abnormal and immature cells should be made. | | |
| • Coagulation Parameters (Non-rodents only):  Bleeding Time, Coagulation Time, Prothrombin Time, Activated Partial Thromboplastin Time | | | |
| Urine analysis Parameters | | | |
| • Colour | • Appearance | • Specific Gravity | • 24-hour urinary output |
| • Reaction (pH) | • Albumin | • Sugar | • Acetone |
| • Bile pigments | • Urobilinogen | • Occult Blood | • Microscopic examination of urinary sediment |
| Blood Biochemical Parameters | | | |
| • Glucose | • Cholesterol | • Triglycerides | • HDL Cholesterol (Non-rodents only) |
| • LDL | • Bilirubin | • SGPT (ALT) | • SGOT (AST) |
| Cholesterol (Non-rodents only) | | | |
| • Alkaline Phosphatase (ALP) | • GGT (Non-rodents only) | • Blood Urea Nitrogen | • Creatinine |
| • Total Proteins | • Albumin | • Globulin (Calculated values) | • Sodium |
| • Potassium | • Phosphorus | • Calcium | |
| Gross and Microscopic Pathology | | | |
| • Brain*: Cerebrum, Cerebellum, Midbrain | • (Spinal Cord) | • Eye | • (Middle Ear) |
| • Thyroid | • (Parathyroid) | • Spleen* | • Thymus |
| • Adrenal* | • (Pancreas) | • (Trachea) | • Lung* |
| • Heart* | • Aorta | • Oesophagus | • Stomach |
| • Duodenum | • Jejunum | • Terminal ileum | • Colon |
| • (Rectum) | • Liver* | • Kidney* | • Urinary bladder |

| • Epididymis | • Testis* | • Ovary | • Uterus* |
|---|---|---|---|
| • Skin | • Mammary gland | • Mesenteric lymph node | • Skeletal muscle |
| * Organs marked with an asterisk should be weighed. | | | |
| () Organs listed in parenthesis should be examined if indicated by the nature of the drug or observed effects. | | | |

Non-clinical toxicity testing and safety evaluation data of an IND needed for the conduct of different phases of clinical trials.

**Note:** Refer Appendix III (Points 1.1 through 1.7 and tables 1.8 and 1.9) for essential features of study designs of the non-clinical toxicity studies listed below.

## For Phase I Clinical Trials

Systemic Toxicity studies

   (i)   Single dose toxicity studies

   (ii)  Dose Ranging Studies

   (iii) Repeat-dose systemic toxicity studies of appropriate duration to support the duration of proposed human exposure.

## Male Fertility Study

### *In-vitro* Genotoxicity Tests

Relevant local toxicity studies with proposed route of clinical application (duration depending on proposed length of clinical exposure)

Allergenicity/Hypersensitivity tests (when there is a cause for concern or for parenteral drugs, including dermal application)

Photo-allergy or dermal photo-toxicity test (if the drug or a metabolite is related to an agent causing photosensitivity or the nature of action suggests such a potential)

## For Phase II Clinical Trials

Provide a summary of all the non-clinical safety data (listed above) already submitted while obtaining the permissions for Phase I trial, with appropriate references.

In case of an application for directly starting a Phase II trial - complete details of the non- clinical safety data needed for obtaining the permission for Phase I trial, as per the list provided above must be submitted.

Repeat-dose systemic toxicity studies of appropriate duration to support the duration of proposed human exposure

In-vivo genotoxicity tests

Segment II reproductive/developmental toxicity study (if female patients of child bearing age are going to be involved)

## For Phase III Clinical Trials

Provide a summary of all the non-clinical safety data (listed above) already submitted while obtaining the permissions for Phase I and II trials, with appropriate references.

In case of an application for directly initiating a Phase III trial - complete details of the non-clinical safety data needed for obtaining the permissions for Phase I and II trials, as per the list provided above must be provided.

Repeat-dose systemic toxicity studies of appropriate duration to support the duration of proposed human exposure

Reproductive/developmental toxicity studies

Segment I (if female patients of child bearing age are going to be involved), and

Segment III (for drugs to be given to pregnant or nursing mothers or where there are indications of possible adverse effects on foetal development).

Carcinogenicity studies (when there is a cause for concern or when the drug is to be used for more than 6 months).

## For Phase IV Clinical Trials

Provide a summary of all the non-clinical safety data (listed above) already submitted while obtaining the permissions for Phase I, II and III trials, with appropriate references.

In case an application is made for initiating the Phase IV trial, complete details of the non-clinical safety data needed for obtaining the permissions for Phase I, II and III trials, as per the list provided above must be submitted.

## Application of Good Laboratory Practices (GLP)

The animal studies must be conducted in an accredited laboratory.

## ANIMAL PHARMACOLOGY

1. **General Principles:** Specific and general pharmacological studies should be conducted to support use of therapeutics in humans. In the early stages of drug development enough information may not be available to rationally select study design for safety assessment. In such a situation, a general approach to safety pharmacology studies can be applied. Safety pharmacology studies are studies that investigate potential undesirable pharmacodynamic effects of a substance on physiological functions in relation to exposure within the therapeutic range or above.

   **1.1 Specific Pharmacological Actions:** Specific pharmacological actions are those which demonstrate the therapeutic potential for humans. The specific studies that should be conducted and their design will be different, based on the individual properties and intended uses of investigational drug. Scientifically validated methods should be used. The use of new technologies and methodologies in accordance with sound scientific principles should be preferred.

   **1.2 General Pharmacological Actions**

   **1.2.1 Essential Safety Pharmacology:** Safety pharmacology studies need to be conducted to investigate the potential undesirable pharmacodynamic effects of a substance on physiological functions in relation to exposure within the therapeutic range and above. These studies should be designed to identify undesirable pharmacodynamic properties of a substance that may have relevance to its human safety; to evaluate adverse pharmacodynamic and/or pathophysiological effects observed in toxicology and/or clinical studies; and to investigate the mechanism of the adverse pharmacodynamic effects observed and/or suspected. The aim of the essential safety pharmacology is to study the effects of the test drug on vital functions. Vital organ systems such as cardiovascular, respiratory and central nervous systems should be studied. Essential safety pharmacology studies may be excluded or supplemented based on scientific rationale. Also, the exclusion of certain test(s) or exploration(s) of certain organs, systems or functions should be scientifically justified.

**1.2.1.1 Cardiovascular System:** Effects of the investigational drug should be studied on blood pressure, heart rate, and the electrocardiogram. If possible *in vitro, in vivo* and/or *ex vivo* methods including electrophysiology should also be considered.

**1.2.1.2 Central Nervous System:** Effects of the investigational drug should be studied on motor activity, behavioral changes, coordination, sensory and motor reflex responses and body temperature.

**1.2.1.3 Respiratory System:** Effects of the investigational drug on respiratory rate and other functions such as tidal volume and heamoglobin oxygen saturation should be studied.

**1.3 Follow-up and Supplemental Safety Pharmacology Studies**: In addition to the essential safety pharmacological studies, additional supplemental and follow-up safety pharmacology studies may need to be conducted as appropriate. These depend on the pharmacological properties or chemical class of the test substance, and the data generated from safety pharmacology studies, clinical trials, pharmacovigilance, experimental *in vitro* or *in vivo* studies, or from literature reports.

**1.3.1 Follow-up Studies For Essential Safety Pharmacology:** Follow-up studies provide additional information or a better understanding than that provided by the essential safety pharmacology.

**1.3.1.1 Cardiovascular System:** These include ventricular contractility, vascular resistance and the effects of chemical mediators, their agonists and antagonists on the cardiovascular system.

**1.3.1.2 Central Nervous System:** These include behavioral studies, learning and memory, electrophysiological studies, neuro-chemistry and ligand binding studies.

**1.3.1.3 Respiratory System:** These include airway resistance, compliance, pulmonary arterial pressure, blood gases and blood pH.

**1.3.2 Supplemental Safety Pharmacology Studies:** These studies are required to investigate the possible adverse pharmacological effects that are not assessed in the essential safety pharmacological studies and are a cause for concern.

**1.3.2.1 Urinary System:** These include urine volume, specific gravity, osmolality, pH, proteins, cytology and blood urea nitrogen, creatinine and plasma proteins estimation.

**1.3.2.2 Autonomic Nervous System:** These include binding to receptors relevant for the autonomic nervous system, and functional response to agonist or antagonist responses *in vivo* or *in vitro*, and effects of direct stimulation of autonomic nerves and their effects on cardiovascular responses.

**1.3.2.3 Gastrointestinal System:** These include studies on gastric secretion, gastric pH measurement, gastric mucosal examination, bile secretion, gastric emptying time *in vivo* and ileocaecal contraction *in vitro*.

**1.3.2.4 Other Organ Systems:** Effects of the investigational drug on organ systems not investigated elsewhere should be assessed when there is a cause for concern. For example dependency potential, skeletal muscle, immune and endocrine functions may be investigated.

**1.4 Conditions Under Which Safety Pharmacology Studies Are Not Necessary:** Safety pharmacology studies are usually not required for locally applied agents e.g. dermal or ocular, in cases when the pharmacology of the investigational drug is well known, and/or when systemic absorption from the site of application is low. Safety pharmacology testing is also not necessary, in case of a new derivative having similar pharmacokinetics and pharmacodynamics.

### 1.5 Timing of Safety Pharmacology Studies in Relation to Clinical Development:

**1.5.1 Prior to First Administration in Humans:** The effects of an investigational drug on the vital functions listed in the essential safety pharmacology should be studied prior to first administration in humans. Any follow-up or supplemental studies identified, should be conducted if necessary, based on a cause for concern.

**1.5.2 During Clinical Development:** Additional investigations may be warranted to clarify observed or suspected adverse effects in animals and humans during clinical development

**1.5.3 Before Applying for Marketing Approval:** Follow-up and supplemental safety pharmacology studies should be assessed prior to approval unless not required, in which case this should be justified. Available information from toxicology studies addressing safety pharmacology endpoints or information from clinical studies can replace such studies.

### 1.6 Application of Good Laboratory Practices (GLP): The animal studies phase must be conducted in an accredited laboratory.

## INFORMED CONSENT

**1.  Checklist for Study Subject's Informed Consent Documents**

**1.1  Essential Elements**

1. Statement that the study involves research and explanation of the purpose of the research

2. Expected duration of the Subject's participation

3. Description of the procedures to be followed, including all invasive procedures.

4. Description of any reasonably foreseeable risks or discomforts to the Subject

5. Description of any benefits to the Subject or others reasonably expected from research. If no benefit is expected Subject should be made aware of this.

6. Disclosure of specific appropriate alternative procedures or therapies available to the Subject.

7. Statement describing the extent to which confidentiality of records identifying the Subject will be maintained and who will have access to Subject's medical records

8. Trial treatment schedule(s) and the probability for random assignment to each treatment (for randomized trials)

9. Statement describing the financial compensation and medical management as under:- (a) In the event of an injury occurring to the clinical trial subject, such subject shall be provided free medical management as long as required. (b) In the event of a trial related injury or death, the Sponsor or his representative, whomsoever has obtained permission from the Licensing Authority for conduct of the clinical trial shall provide financial compensation for the injury or death.

10. An explanation about whom to contact for trial related queries, rights of Subjects and in the event of any injury

11. The anticipated prorated payment, if any, to be given to the Subject for participating in the trial

12. Subject's responsibilities on participation in the trial

13. Statement that participation is voluntary, that the subject can withdraw from the study at any time and that refusal to participate will not involve any penalty or loss of benefits to which the Subject is otherwise entitled

14. Any other pertinent information

## 1.2 Additional Elements, which may be required

1. Statement of foreseeable circumstances under which the Subject's participation may be terminated by the Investigator without the Subject's consent.

2. Additional costs to the Subject that may result from participation in the study.

3. The consequences of a Subject's decision to withdraw from the research and procedures for orderly termination of participation by Subject.

4. Statement that the Subject or Subject's representative will be notified in a timely manner if significant new findings develop during the course of the research which may affect the Subject's willingness to continue participation will be provided.

5. A statement that the particular treatment or procedure may involve risks to the Subject (or to the embryo or fetus, if the Subject is or may become pregnant), which are currently unforeseeable

6. Approximate number of Subjects enrolled in the study

**2.    Format of Informed Consent form for Subjects Participating in a Clinical Trial**

Informed Consent form to participate in a clinical trial

Study Title:

Study Number:

Subject's Initials:                    Date of Birth / Age:

Address of the subject ...............

Subject's Name:

Qualification .......................... Occupation:

Student/Self-Employed/Service/Housewife/Others    (Please    tick    as appropriate)

Annual Income of the subject ............

Name and address of the nominee(s) and his relation to the subject ............ (for the purpose of compensation in case of trial related death).

Please initial box (Subject)

- (i)    I confirm that I have read and understood the information sheet dated _for the above study and have had the opportunity to ask questions. [ ]
- (ii)   I understand that my participation in the study is voluntary and that I am free to withdraw at any time, without giving any reason, without my medical care or legal rights being affected. [ ]
- (iii)  I understand that the Sponsor of the clinical trial, others working on the Sponsor's behalf, the Ethics Committee and the regulatory authorities will not need my permission to look at my health records both in respect of the current study and any further research that may be conducted in relation to it, even if I withdraw from the trial. I agree to this access. However, I understand that my identity will not be revealed in any information released to third parties or published. [ ]
- (iv)   I agree not to restrict the use of any data or results that arise from this study, provided such a use is only for scientific purpose(s) [ ]
- (v)    I agree to take part in the above study. [ ]

Date: /_ /

Signature (or Thumb impression) of the Subject/Legally   Acceptable
Representative:                    Signatory's                    Name:

_________________________________________________________________

Signature                of                the                Investigator:
Date: _ / _/

Study Investigator 's Name: _

Signature              of              the              Witness              _
Date: / /

Name of the Witness: _ _ _ _ _ _

[Copy of the Patient Information Sheet and duly filled Informed Consent
Form shall be handed over to the subject or his/her attendant.]

## FIXED DOSE COMBINATIONS (FDCs)

Fixed Dose Combinations refer to products containing one or more active ingredients used for a particular indication(s). FDCs can be divided into the following groups and data required for approval for marketing is described below:

(a) The first group of FDCs includes those in which one or more of the active ingredients is a new drug. For such FDCs to be approved for marketing data to be submitted will be similar to data required for any new drug (including clinical trials) [see rule 122E, item (a)].

(b) The second group FDCs includes those in which active ingredients already approved/ marketed individually are combined for the first time, for a particular claim and where the ingredients are likely to have significant interaction of a pharmacodynamic or pharmacokinetic nature [see rule 122E, item (c)]. If clinical trials have been carried out with the FDC in other countries, reports of such trials should be submitted. If the FDC is marketed abroad, the regulatory status in other countries should be stated. (see Appendix I, item 9).

(i) For marketing permission, appropriate chemical and pharmaceutical data will be submitted. In case, such a combination is not marketed anywhere in the world but these drugs are already in use concomitantly (not as an FDC but individually) for the said claim, marketing permission may be granted based on chemical and pharmaceutical data. Data showing the stability of the proposed dosage form will also have to be submitted.

(ii) For any other such FDCs, clinical trials may be required. For obtaining permission to carry out clinical trials with such FDCs a summary of available pharmacological, toxicological and clinical data on the individual ingredients should be submitted, along with the rationale for combining them in the proposed ratio. In addition, acute toxicity data ($LD_{50}$) and pharmacological data should be submitted on the individual ingredients as well as their combination in the proposed ratio.

(c) The third group of FDCs includes those which are already marketed, but in which it is proposed either to change the ratio of active ingredients or to make a new therapeutic claim. For such FDCs, the appropriate rationale including published reports (if any) should be submitted to obtain marketing permission. Permission will be granted depending upon the nature of the claim and data submitted.

(d) The fourth group of FDC includes those whose individual active ingredients (or drugs from the same class) have been widely used in a particular indication(s) for years, their concomitant use is often necessary and no claim is proposed to be made other than convenience. It will have to be demonstrated that the proposed dosage form is stable and the ingredients are unlikely to have significant interaction of a pharmacodynamic or pharmacokinetic nature.

No additional animal or human data are generally required for these FDCs, and marketing permission may be granted if the FDC has an acceptable rationale.

## UNDERTAKING BY THE INVESTIGATOR

1. Full name, address and title of the Principal Investigator (or Investigator(s) when there is no Principal Investigator)

2. Name and address of the medical college, hospital or other facility where the clinical trial will be conducted: Education, training & experience that qualify the Investigator for the clinical trial (Attach details including Medical Council registration number, and / or any other statement(s) of qualification(s))

3. Name and address of all clinical laboratory facilities to be used in the study.

4. Name and address of the Ethics Committee that is responsible for approval and continuing review of the study.

5. Names of the other members of the research team (Co- or sub-Investigators) who will be assisting the Investigator in the conduct of the investigation (s).

6. Protocol Title and Study number (if any) of the clinical trial to be conducted by the Investigator.

7. Commitments:

    (i)    I have reviewed the clinical protocol and agree that it contains all the necessary information to conduct the study. I will not begin the study until all necessary Ethics Committee and regulatory approvals have been obtained.

    (ii)    I agree to conduct the study in accordance with the current protocol. I will not implement any deviation from or changes of the protocol without agreement by the Sponsor and prior review and documented approval / favorable opinion from the Ethics Committee of the amendment, except where necessary to eliminate an immediate hazard(s) to the trial Subjects or when the change(s) involved are only logistical or administrative in nature.

(iii) I agree to personally conduct and/or supervise the clinical trial at my site.

(iv) I agree to inform all Subjects, that the drugs are being used for investigational purposes and I will ensure that the requirements relating to obtaining informed consent and ethics committee review and approval specified in the GCP guidelines are met.

(v) I agree to report to the Sponsor all adverse experiences that occur in the course of the investigation(s) in accordance with the regulatory and GCP guidelines.

(vi) I have read and understood the information in the Investigator's brochure, including the potential risks and side effects of the drug.

(vii) I agree to ensure that all associates, colleagues and employees assisting in the conduct of the study are suitably qualified and experienced and they have been informed about their obligations in meeting their commitments in the trial.

(viii) I agree to maintain adequate and accurate records and to make those records available for audit / inspection by the Sponsor, Ethics Committee, Licensing Authority or their authorized representatives, in accordance with regulatory and GCP provisions. I will fully cooperate with any study related audit conducted by regulatory officials or authorized representatives of the Sponsor.

(ix) I agree to promptly report to the Ethics Committee all changes in the clinical trial activities and all unanticipated problems involving risks to human Subjects or others.

(x) I agree to inform all unexpected serious adverse events to the Sponsor as well as the Ethics Committee within seven days of their occurence.

(xi)  I will maintain confidentiality of the identification of all participating study patients and assure security and confidentiality of study data.

(xii)  I agree to comply with all other requirements, guidelines and statutory obligations as applicable to clinical Investigators participating in clinical trials.

8.  Signature of the Investigator with Date.

## ETHICS COMMITTEE INCLUDING REGISTRATION

### I. Requirements and Guidelines for Registration of Ethics Committee

1. **Scope:** Ethics Committee shall review every clinical trial proposal and evaluate the possible risks to the subjects, expected benefits and adequacy of documentation for ensuring privacy, confidentiality and justice. In the case of any serious adverse event occurring to the clinical trial subjects during the clinical trial, the Ethics Committee shall analyze and forward its opinion as per procedures specified in APPENDIX XII of Schedule Y.

2. **Composition of Ethics Committee:**

   (a) Ethics Committee shall consist of not less than seven members and one among its members, who is from outside the institute, shall be appointed as Chairman; one member as a Member Secretary and rest of the members shall be from Medical, Scientific, Non-medical and Non-scientific fields including lay public.

   (b) The committee shall include at least one member whose primary area of interest or specialization is Non-scientific and at least one member who is independent of the institution. Besides, there should be appropriate gender representation on the Ethics Committee.

   (c) The Ethics Committee can have as its members, individuals from other Institutions or Communities, if required.

   (d) Members should be conversant with the provisions of clinical trials under this Schedule, Good Clinical Practice Guidelines for clinical trials in India and other regulatory requirements to safeguard the rights, safety and well- being of the trial subjects.

   (e) For review of each protocol the quorum of Ethics Committee shall be at least five members with the following representations:

   - Basic medical scientist (preferably one pharmacologist);

- Clinician;
- Legal expert;
- Social Scientist or representative of non-governmental voluntary agency or philosopher or ethicist or theologian or a similar person;
- Lay person from the community.

(f)  The members representing medical scientists and clinicians should have post graduate qualification and adequate experience in their respective fields and must be aware of their roles and responsibilities as committee members.

(g)  As far as possible, based on the requirement of research area such as HIV, Genetic disorder etc., specific patient group may also be represented in the Ethics Committee.

(h)  There should be no conflict of interest. The members shall voluntarily withdraw from the Ethics Committee meeting while making a decision on an application which evokes a conflict of interest which may be indicated in writing to the Chairman prior to the review and be recorded so in the minutes. All members shall sign a declaration on conflict of interest.

(i)  Subject experts or other experts may be invited to the meetings for their advice. But no such expert shall have voting rights.

**3. Information required to be Submitted by the Applicant for Registration of Ethics Committee:**

(a)  Name of the Ethics Committee

(b)  Authority under which the Ethics Committee has been constituted, membership requirements, the term of reference, conditions of appointment and the quorum required.

(c)  The procedure for resignation, replacement or removal of members.

(d)  Address of the office of the Ethics Committee.

(e)  Name, address, qualification, organizational title, telephone number, fax number, email, mailing address and brief profile of the Chairman.

(f)  Names, qualifications, organizational title, telephone number, fax number, e-mail and mailing address of the members of the Ethics Committee. The information shall also include member's specialty (primary, scientific or non - scientific), member's affiliation with institutions and patient group representation, if any.

(g) Details of the supporting staff.

(h) In the case of Ethics Committees existing before the publication of the Drugs and Cosmetics (Third Amendment) Rules, 2013,

- Type of clinical research reviewed by the committee (e.g. pharmaceuticals, devices, epidemiological, retrospective, herbals, etc.)

- Documents reviewed for every clinical trial protocol including Informed Consent documents.

- Information in respect of number of meetings of the committee and documentation of the minutes of meetings of these committees concerning clinical trials.

- Information regarding review of serious adverse events reported during the conduct of the trial.

(i) The Standard Operating Procedures to be followed by the committee in general.

(j). Standard Operating Procedures to be followed by the committee for vulnerable population.

(k) Policy regarding training for new and existing committee members along with Standard Operating Procedures.

(l) Policy to monitor or prevent the conflict of interest along with Standard Operating Procedures.

(m) If the committee has been audited or inspected before, give details.

4. **Maintenance of Record**: All documentation and communication of an Ethics Committee are to be dated, filed and preserved according to the Standard Operating Procedures. Strict confidentiality shall be maintained during access and retrieval procedures. Records should be maintained for the following, namely:-

(a) The constitution and composition of the Ethics Committee;

(b) The curriculum vitae of all the committee members;

(c) Standard Operating Procedures followed by the committee;

(d) National and international guidelines;

(e) Copies of the protocol, data collection formats, Case Report Forms, Investigator's brochures, etc, submitted for review;

(f) All correspondence with committee members and Investigators regarding application, decision and follow up;

(g) Agenda of all Ethics Committee meetings;

(h) Minutes of all Ethics Committee meetings with signature of the Chairman;

(i) Copies of decisions communicated to the applicants;

(j) Record of all notification issued for premature termination of a study with a summary of the reasons;

(k) Final report of the study including microfilms, compact disks or video-recordings. All records shall be safely maintained after the completion or termination of the study for not less than five years from the date of completion or termination of the trial (Both in hard and soft copies).

5. **The Ethics Committee shall be Open to Inspection** by the officers authorized by the Central Drugs Standard Control Organization, who may include an officer of the State Drug Control Authority concerned, to verify compliance to the requirements of Schedule Y, Good Clinical Practice guidelines and other applicable regulation for safeguarding the rights, safety and well-being of the trial subjects.

II. **Format for According Approval to Clinical Trial protocol by the Ethics Committee**

To

Dr.

Dear Dr.

The Institutional Ethics Committee / Independent Ethics Committee (state name of the committee, as appropriate) reviewed and discussed your application to conduct the clinical trial entitled "......" on .......(date).

*The following documents were reviewed:*

(a) Trial Protocol (including protocol amendments), dated _ Version no (s).___________

(b) Patient Information Sheet and Informed Consent Form (including updates if any) in English and/or vernacular language.

(c) Investigator's Brochure, dated _        , Version no.

(d) Proposed methods for patient accrual including advertisement (s) etc. proposed to be used for the purpose.

(e) Principal Investigator's current CV.

(f) Insurance Policy / Compensation for participation and for serious adverse events occurring during the study participation.

(g) Investigator's Agreement with the Sponsor.

(h) Investigator's Undertaking (Appendix VII).

The following members of the ethics committee were present at the meeting held on (date, time, place).

-------------------------------Chairman of the Ethics Committee

----------------------------------Member secretary of the Ethics Committee

-------------------------- Name of each member with designation

We approve the trial to be conducted in its presented form. The Institutional Ethics Committee / Independent Ethics Committee expects to be informed  about the progress of the study, any SAE occurring in the course of the study, any changes in the protocol and patient information/informed consent and asks to be provided  a copy of the final report.

Yours sincerely,

Member Secretary, Ethics Committee.

## STABILITY TESTING OF NEW DRUGS

Stability testing is to be performed to provide evidence on how the quality of a drug substance or formulation varies with time under the influence of various environmental factors such as temperature, humidity and light, and to establish shelf life for the formulation and recommended storage conditions.

Stability studies should include testing of those attributes of the drug substance that are susceptible to change during storage and are likely to influence quality, safety, and/or efficacy. In case of formulations the testing should cover, as appropriate, the physical, chemical, biological, and microbiological attributes, preservative content (e.g., antioxidant, antimicrobial preservative), and functionality tests (e.g., for a dose delivery system).

Validated stability-indicating analytical procedures should be applied. For long term studies, frequency of testing should be sufficient to establish the stability profile of the drug substance.

In general, a drug substance should be evaluated under storage conditions that tests its thermal stability and, if applicable, its sensitivity to moisture. The storage conditions and the length of studies chosen should be sufficient to cover storage, shipment and subsequent use.

Stress testing of the drug substance should be conducted to identify the likely degradation products, which in turn establishes the degradation pathways, evaluates the intrinsic stability of the molecule and validates the stability indicating power of the analytical procedures used. The nature of the stress testing will depend on the individual drug substance and the type of formulation involved.

Stress testing may generally be carried out on a single batch of the drug substance. It should include the effect of temperatures, humidity where appropriate, oxidation, and photolysis on the drug substance.

*Data should be provided for:*

(a) Photostability on at least one primary batch of the drug substance as well as the formulation, as the case may be and

(b) The susceptibility of the drug substance to hydrolysis across a wide range of pH values when in solution or suspension.

Long-term testing should cover a minimum of 12 months' duration on at least three primary batches of the drug substance or the formulation at the time of submission and should be continued for a period of time sufficient to cover the proposed shelf life. Accelerated testing should cover a minimum of 6 months duration at the time of submission. In case of drug substances, the batches should be manufactured to a minimum of pilot scale by the same synthetic route and using a method of manufacture that simulates the final process to be used for production batches.

In case of formulations, two of the three batches should be at least pilot scale and the third one may be smaller. The manufacturing process(es) used for primary batches should simulate that to be applied to production batches and should provide products of the same quality and meeting the same specifications as that intended for marketing. The stability studies for drug substances should be conducted either in the same container - closure system as proposed for storage and distribution or in a container - closure system that simulates the proposed final packaging. In case of formulations, the stability studies should be conducted in the final container - closure system proposed for marketing.

***Stability Testing of new drug substances and formulations:***

(i) **Study conditions for drug substances and formulations intended to be stored under general conditions**

| Study | Study conditions | Duration of study |
| --- | --- | --- |
| Long term | $30°C \pm 2°C/65\%$ RH $\pm 5\%$ RH | 12 months |
| Accelerated | $40°C \pm 2°C/75\%$ RH $\pm 5\%$ RH | 6 months |

If at any time during 6 months' testing under the accelerated storage condition, such changes occur that cause the product to fail in complying with the prescribed standards, additional testing under an intermediate storage condition should be conducted and evaluated against significant change criteria.

(ii) **Study conditions for drug substances and formulations intended to be stored in a refrigerator**

| Study | Study conditions | Duration of study |
| --- | --- | --- |
| Long term | $5°C \pm 3°C$ | 12 months |
| Accelerated | $25°C \pm 2°C/60\%$ RH $\pm 5\%$ RH | 6 months |

(iii) **Study conditions for drug substances and formulations intended to be stored in a freezer Study**

| **Study** | **conditions** | **Duration of study** |
|---|---|---|
| Long term | - 20°C ± 5°C | 12 months |

(iv) **Drug substances intended for storage below -20°C** shall be treated on a case-by-case basis.

(v) **Stability testing of the formulation after constitution or dilution**, if applicable, should be conducted to provide information for the labelling on the preparation, storage condition, and in-use period of the constituted or diluted product. This testing should be performed on the constituted or diluted product through the proposed in-use period.

# APPENDIX - X

## CONTENTS OF THE PROPOSED PROTOCOL FOR CONDUCTING CLINICAL TRIALS

1. **Title Page**

   (a) Full title of the clinical study,

   (b) Protocol/Study number, and protocol version number with date

   (c) The IND name/number of the investigational drug

   (d) Complete name and address of the Sponsor and contract research organization if any

   (e) List of the Investigators who are conducting the study, their respective institutional affiliations and site locations

   (f) Name(s) of clinical laboratories and other departments and/or facilities participating in the study.

2. **Table of Contents:** A complete table of contents including a list of all Appendices.

2.1. **Background and Introduction**

   (a) Preclinical experience.

   (b) Clinical experience.

Previous clinical work with the new drug should be reviewed here and a description of how the current protocol extends existing data should be provided. If this is an entirely new indication, how this drug was considered for this should be discussed. Relevant information regarding pharmacological, toxicological and other biological properties of the drug/biologic/ medical device, and previous efficacy and safety experience should be described.

2.2 **Study Rationale:** This section should describe a brief summary of the background information relevant to the study design and protocol methodology. The reasons for performing this study in the particular population included by the protocol should be provided.

**2.3.** **Study Objective(s) (primary as well as secondary) and their logical relation to the study design.**

**2.4.** **Study Design**

(a) Overview of the Study Design: Including a description of the type of study (i.e., double-blind, multicentre, placebo controlled, etc.), a detail of the specific treatment groups and number of study Subjects in each group and investigative site, Subject number assignment, the type, sequence and duration of study periods.

(b) Flow chart of the study

(c) A brief description of the methods and procedures to be used during the study.

(d) Discussion of Study Design: This discussion details the rationale for the design chosen for this study.

**2.5.** **Study Population:** the number of Subjects required to be enrolled in the study at the investigative site and by all sites along with a brief description of the nature of the Subject population required is also mentioned.

**2.6.** **Subject Eligibility**

(a) Inclusion Criteria

(b) Exclusion Criteria

**2.7.** **Study Assessments** – plan, procedures and methods to be described in detail

**2.8.** **Study Conduct** stating the types of study activities that would be included in this section would be: medical history, type of physical examination, blood or urine testing, electrocardiogram (ECG), diagnostic testing such as pulmonary function tests, symptom measurement, dispensation and retrieval of medication, Subject cohort assignment, adverse event review, etc.

Each visit should be described separately as Visit 1, Visit 2, etc.

**Discontinued Subjects**: Describes the circumstances for Subject withdrawal, dropouts, or other reasons for discontinuation of Subjects. State how dropouts would be managed and if they would be replaced. Describe the method of handling of protocol waivers, if any. The person(s) who approves all such waivers should be identified and the criteria used for specific waivers should be provided.

Describe how protocol violations will be treated, including conditions where the study will be terminated for non-compliance with the protocol.

### 2.9. Study Treatment

(a) Dosing schedule (dose, frequency, and duration of the experimental treatment) Describe the administration of placebos and/or dummy medications if they are part of the treatment plan. If applicable, concomitant drug(s), their doses, frequency, and duration of concomitant treatment should be stated.

(b) Study drug supplies and administration: A statement about who is going to provide the study medication and that the investigational drug formulation has been manufactured following all regulations, Details of the product stability, storage requirements and dispensing requirements should be provided.

(c) Dose modification for studing of drug toxicity: Rules for changing the dose or stopping the study drug should be provided.

(d) Possible drug interactions.

(e) Concomitant therapy: The drugs that are permitted during the study and the conditions under which they may be used are detailed here. Describe the drugs that a Subject is not allowed to use during parts of or the entire study. If any washout periods for prohibited medications are needed prior to enrolment, these should be described here.

(f) Blinding procedures: A detailed description of the blinding procedure if the study employs a blind on the Investigator and/or the Subject.

(g) Unblinding procedures: If the study is blinded, the circumstances in which unblinding may be done and the mechanism to be used for unblinding should be given.

**2.10** **Adverse Events** (See Appendix XI): Description of expected adverse events should be given. Procedures used to evaluate an adverse event should be described.

**2.11. Ethical Considerations**: Give the summary of:

(a) Risk/benefit assessment.

(b) Ethics Committee review and communications.

(c) Informed consent process.

(d) Statement of Subject confidentiality including ownership of data and coding procedures.

**2.12. Study Monitoring and Supervision:** A description of study monitoring policies and procedures should be provided along with the proposed frequency of site monitoring visits, and who is expected to perform monitoring. Case Record Form (CRF) completion requirements, including who gets which copies of the forms and any specifics required in filling out the forms CRF correction requirements, including who is authorized to make corrections on the CRF and how queries about study data are handled and how errors, if any, are to be corrected should be stated. Investigator study files, including what needs to be stored following study completion should be described.

**2.13. Investigational Product Management**

(a) Give Investigational product description and packaging (stating all Ingredients and the formulation of the investigational drug and any placebos used in the study)

(b) The precise dosing required during the study.

(c) Method of packaging, labelling, and blinding of study substances.

(d) Method of assigning treatments to Subjects and the Subject identification code numbering system.

(e) Storage conditions for study substances.

(f) Investigational product accountability: Describe instructions for the receipt, storage, dispensation, and return of the investigational products to ensure a complete accounting of all investigational products received, dispensed, and returned/destroyed.

(g.) Describe policy and procedure for handling unused investigational products.

**2.14. Data Analysis:** Provide details of the statistical approach to be followed including sample size, how the sample size was determined, including assumptions made in making this determination, efficacy endpoints (primary as well as secondary) and safety endpoints.

**Statistical analysis:** Give complete details of how the results will be analyzed and reported along with the description of statistical tests to be used to analyze the primary and secondary endpoints defined above. Describe the level of significance, statistical tests to be used, and the methods used for missing data; method of evaluation of the data for treatment failures, non- compliance, and Subject withdrawals; rationale and conditions for any interim analysis if planned.

Describe statistical considerations for Pharmacokinetic (PK) analysis, if applicable.

**2.15.** **Undertaking by the Investigator** (see Appendix VII).

**2.16.** **Appendices**: Provide a study synopsis, copies of the informed consent documents (patient information sheet, informed consent form etc.); CRF and other data collection forms; a summary of relevant pre-clinical safety information and any other documents referenced in the clinical protocol.

## DATA ELEMENTS FOR REPORTING SERIOUS ADVERSE EVENTS OCCURING IN A CLINICAL TRIAL

1. **Patient Details:** Initials & other relevant identifier (hospital/OPD record number etc.)*

   Gender

   Age and/or date of birth

   Weight

   Height

2. **Suspected Drug (s)**

   Generic name of the drug*

   Indication(s) for which suspect drug was prescribed or tested

   Dosage form and strength

   Daily dose and regimen (specify units - e.g., mg, ml, mg/kg)

   Route of administration

   Starting date and time of day

   Stopping date and time, or duration of treatment

3. **Other Treatment (s):** Provide the same information for concomitant drugs (including non prescription/OTC drugs) and non-drug therapies, as for the suspected drug(s).

4. **Details of Suspected Adverse Drug Reaction(s):** Full description of reaction(s) including body site and severity, as well as the criterion (or criteria) for regarding the report as serious. In addition to a description of the reported signs and symptoms, whenever possible, describe a specific diagnosis for the reaction*

   Start date (and time) of onset of reaction

   Stop date (and time) or duration of reaction

Dechallenge and rechallenge information

Setting (e.g., hospital, out-patient clinic, home, nursing home)

## 5. Outcome

Information on recovery and any sequelae; results of specific tests and/or treatment that may have been conducted.

For a fatal outcome, cause of death and a comment on its possible relationship to the suspected reaction; any post-mortem findings.

**Other information:** Anything relevant to facilitate assessment of the case, such as medical history including allergy, drug or alcohol abuse; family history; findings from special investigations etc.

## 6. Details about the Investigator*

Name

Address

Telephone number

Profession (speciality)

Date of reporting the event to Licensing Authority

Date of reporting the event to Ethics Committee overseeing the site

Signature of the Investigator

**Note: Information marked * must be provided.**

## COMPENSATION IN CASE OF INJURY OR DEATH DURING CLINICAL TRIAL

1. In the case of an injury occurring to the clinical trial subject, he or she shall be given free medical management as long as required.

2. In case the injury occurring to the trial subject is related to the clinical trial, such subject shall also be entitled for financial compensation as per order of the Licensing Authority defined under clause (b) of Rule 21 and the financial compensation will be over and above any expenses incurred on the medical management of the subject.

3. In the case of clinical trial related death of the subject, his/her nominee(s) would be entitled for financial compensation as per the order of the Licensing Authority defined under clause (b) of Rule 21, and the financial compensation will be over and above any expenses incurred on the medical management of the subject.

4. The financial compensation for clinical trial related injury or death could be in the form of :-

    (a)    Payment for medical management;

    (b)    Financial compensation for trail related injury;

    (c)    Financial compensation to nominee(s) of the trial subject in case of death;

    (d)    Financial compensation for the child injured in –utero because of the participation of parent in clinical trial.

5. The Sponsor or his representative, whosoever had obtained permission from the Licensing Authority for conduct of the clinical trial shall provide financial compensation, if the injury or death has occurred because of any or the following reasons, namely:-

    (a)    Adverse effect of investigational product(s);

    (b)    Any clinical trial procedures involved in the study;

    (c)    Violation of the approved protocol, scientific misconduct or negligence by the Sponsor or his representative or the Investigator;

    (d)    Failure of investigational product to provide intended therapeutic effect;

    (e)    Use of placebo in a placebo controlled trial;

    (f)    Adverse effects due to concomitant medication excluding standard care, necessitated as part of approved protocol;

    (g)    Injury to the child in-utero because of the participation of parent in clinical trial.

6. Procedure for payment of financial compensation. (a) The Investigator shall report all serious and unexpected adverse events to the Licensing Authority as defined under clause (b) of Rule 21, the Sponsor or his representative whosoever had obtained permission from the Licensing Authority for conduct of the clinical trial and the Ethics Committee that accorded approval to the study protocol, within twenty four hours of their occurrence as per Appendix XI. (b)

(i)    The cases of serious adverse events of death shall be examined as under:

    (A)    An independent Expert Committee shall be constituted by the Licensing Authority as defined under Rule 21(b) to examine the cases and recommend to the Licensing Authority for the purpose of arriving at the cause of death and quantum of compensation in case of clinical trial related death.

    (B)    The Sponsor or his representative, whosoever had obtained permission from the Licensing Authority for conducting the clinical trial and the Investigator shall forward their reports on serious adverse event of death after due analysis to Chairman of the Ethics Committee and Chairman of the Expert Committee with a copy of the report to the Licensing Authority as defined under Rule 21(b) and the head of the Institution where the trial has been conducted within ten calendar days of occurrence of the serious adverse event of death.

    (C)    The Ethics Committee shall forward its report on serious adverse event of death after due analysis along with its opinion on the financial compensation, if any, to be paid by the Sponsor or his representative, whosoever had obtained permission from the Licensing Authority as defined under Rule 21(b) for conducting the clinical trial, to the Chairman of the Expert Committee with a copy of the report to the Licensing Authority within twenty one calendar days of the occurrence of the serious adverse event of death.

(D)    The Expert Committee shall examine the report of serious adverse event of death and give its recommendations to the Licensing Authority for the purpose of arriving at the cause of the adverse event within thirty days of receiving the report from the Ethics Committee, and the expert committee while examining the event, may take into consideration, the reports of the Investigator, Sponsor or his representative whosoever had obtained permission from the Licensing Authority for conducting the clinical trial and the Ethics Committee.

(E)    In the case of clinical trial related death, the Expert Committee shall also recommend the quantum of compensation to be paid by the Sponsor or his representative, whosoever had obtained permission from the Licensing Authority as defined under Rule 21(b) for conducting the clinical trial.

(F)    The Licensing Authority shall consider the recommendations of the Expert Committee and shall determine the cause of death and pass orders as deemed necessary.

(G)    In case of clinical trial related death, the Licensing Authority, after considering the recommendations of the Expert Committee, shall decide the quantum of compensation to be paid by the Sponsor or his representative, whosoever had obtained permission from the Licensing Authority for conducting the clinical trial and shall pass orders as deemed necessary within three months of receiving the report of the serious adverse event.

(ii)    Cases of serious adverse events, other than deaths, shall be examined as under:

(A)    The Sponsor or his representative, whosoever had obtained permission from the Licensing Authority for conducting the clinical trial, and the Investigator shall forward their reports on serious adverse event, after due analysis, to the Licensing Authority as defined under Rule 21(b), Chairman of the Ethics Committee and the head of the Institution where the trial has been conducted within ten calendar days of occurrence of the serious adverse event.

(B) The Ethics Committee shall forward its report on the serious adverse event, after due analysis along with its opinion regarding the financial compensation, if any, to be paid by the Sponsor or his representative, whosoever had obtained permission from the Licensing Authority as defined under Rule 21(b) for conducting the clinical trial, to the Licensing Authority within twenty one calendar days of occurrence of the serious adverse event.

(C) The Licensing Authority shall determine the cause of injury and pass order as deemed necessary. The Licensing Authority shall have the option to constitute an independent Expert Committee, wherever considered necessary, to examine such serious adverse events of injury, which will be recommended to the Licensing Authority for arriving at the cause of the injury and also the quantum of compensation in case of clinical trial related injury, to be paid by the Sponsor or his representative whosoever had obtained permission from the Licensing Authority as defined under Rule 21(b) for conducting the clinical trial.

(D) In case of clinical trial related injury, the Licensing Authority, shall decide the quantum of compensation to be paid by the Sponsor or his representative whosoever had obtained permission from the Licensing Authority for conducting the clinical trial and shall pass orders as deemed necessary within three months of receiving the report of the serious adverse event.

(iii) The sponsor or his representative, whosoever had obtained permission from the Licensing Authority for conducting the clinical trial shall pay the compensation in case of clinical trial related injury or death as per the order of the Licensing Authority as defined under Rule 21(b) within thirty days of the receipt of such order.

# FACTOR (F) FOR CALCULATING THE AMOUNT OF COMPENSATION

| Age in Years [Not more than] | Factor | Age in Years [Not more than] | Factor |
| --- | --- | --- | --- |
| 16 | 228.54 | 42 | 178.49 |
| 17 | 227.49 | 43 | 175.54 |
| 18 | 226.38 | 44 | 172.52 |
| 19 | 225.22 | 45 | 169.44 |
| 20 | 224.00 | 46 | 166.29 |
| 21 | 222.71 | 47 | 163.07 |
| 22 | 221.37 | 48 | 159.80 |
| 23 | 219.95 | 49 | 156.47 |
| 24 | 218.47 | 50 | 153.09 |
| 25 | 216.91 | 51 | 149.67 |
| 26 | 215.28 | 52 | 146.20 |
| 27 | 213.57 | 53 | 142.68 |
| 28 | 211.79 | 54 | 139.13 |
| 29 | 209.92 | 55 | 135.56 |
| 30 | 207.98 | 56 | 131.95 |
| 31 | 205.95 | 57 | 128.33 |
| 32 | 203.85 | 58 | 124.70 |
| 33 | 201.66 | 59 | 121.05 |
| 34 | 199.40 | 60 | 117.41 |
| 35 | 197.06 | 61 | 113.77 |
| 36 | 194.64 | 62 | 110.14 |
| 37 | 192.14 | 63 | 106.52 |
| 38 | 189.56 | 64 | 102.93 |
| 39 | 186.90 | 65 or more | 99.37 |
| 40 | 186.90 | | |

# VOLUNTEER INFORMATION SHEET AND CONSENT FORM

**(This is just an example. It is not claimed as ideal but it can be used as guide)**

| ICF Version: 01 | Version Date: 10 February 2016 |
| --- | --- |
| This is a research study.<br>The following information is important for you.<br>Please read carefully and ask questions if any information is not clear to you. | |
| Subject ID: | Date: |

**STUDY TITLE:** *Single Dose Fasting Bioequivalence Study of XXX (name of the product with strength and manufacturer) to XXX (name of the product with strength and manufacturer)in Healthy Adult Male Volunteers.*

1. **Study Objective:** This is a research study to assess bioequivalence and monitor adverse events, if any, of two medicinal products meant for human use. One product with proven efficacy is already in extensive use (Reference Product) and the other product is new preparation being sought to be introduced into use (Test Product). Both the products contain the same active ingredient in same quantity

    The details of the two products are:

    **Test Product (A):** XXX (Name, Dosage form and Strength; and Manufacturer).

    **Reference Product (B):** XXX (Name, Dosage form and Strength; and Manufacturer).

2. **Description of Medicine:** What is this medicine that you would be taking?

    XXX (*assuming as an antihistamine*) belongs to a group of medicines called antihistamines. It is used to relieve allergic symptoms of seasonal rhinitis including running nose, sneezing, red, itchy, or watery eyes, or itching of nose, throat, or roof of the mouth in adults and children of 2 years and older. It is also used to relive symptoms of urticaria (hives, red, itchy raised areas of the skin) including itching and rash in adults and children of 6 months and older.

XXX is available here as suspension (of strength ---) to be taken by mouth. In this study you will be given 5 ml (*the exact quantity to be specified*) of this suspension along with 240 ml drinking water in each of the periods under fed condition.

You will be given a high fat breakfast before each dosing. The breakfast consists of two slices of bread with 20 gram butter, chicken tikka 75 gram, egg omelette 20 gram, hash brown potatoes 85 gram with 5 gram butter and whole milk 240 millilitre.

**Form of Medicine (Product)**: Oral Suspension.

**Use of this Medicine**:

1. It is used to relieve symptoms associated with seasonal allergic rhinitis in children 2 to 11 years of age. It effectively treats sneezing, rhinorrhea, itchy nose/palate/throat itchy/watery/red eyes.

2. It is also used in the treatment of uncomplicated skin manifestations of chronic idiopathic urticaria (eruption of large itch wheals on the skin of unknown reason) in children 6 months to 11 years of age.

3. **Your Participation in the Study:** You are one of the 16 healthy, adult, human volunteer being recruited to participate in the study. A through medical check up will be done as described below to assess your suitability to participate in this study:

Physical examination

Chest X – ray

ECG

Blood and Urine tests

Hepatitis B and C

HIV

RPR for Syphilis

Urine test for pregnancy (for female volunteers at the time of screening, admission and after completion of the study)

Urine test for traces of habit forming drugs like benzodiazepines, cannabinoids, ethanol, amphetamines, cocaine, barbiturates and opiates. This test will be done at the beginning of each study period.

For the above investigations, adequate blood samples (9 ml) will be collected. First the blood sample will be checked to see if your blood cell status is adequate for you to participate in the study. If the blood cell status is normal, then the remaining blood samples will be sent for further investigation.

In the event of not normal blood cell status, further investigations will not be done. The remaining blood samples will be disposed as per standard procedure usually followed.

In case of any significant abnormalities in the screening parameters, you will not be eligible to participate in this study. However, you are free to discuss these matters with our doctors available in the campus.

If you are found suitable, then you will be enrolled for the study.

4. **Study Description:** There are two periods in this study. Each period is of 48 hours (2 days) duration. There will be gap of 7 days between each period (wash out period). The entire duration of the study will be of at least 16 days.

   In this study, you will receive a single dose of the test product and reference product in different period. The order in which you will receive either test or reference product will be decided on randomization technique

5. **Housing and Stay:** During the study, you will be checking in into our facility at least 11 hours before you take the study medicine and will be housed for at least 48 hours after taking the study medicine.

6. **Your Responsibilities:**
   - You should inform the doctor at our facility if you are allergic to any medicine.
   - You should not use any other medicines, whether prescribed or common medicines available without prescription, within the

past 30 days prior to dosing in the first period and through out the study.

- You should not smoke cigarettes, beedi and consume other tobacco products like gukha, khaini etc. for at least 48 hours (2days) before the start of each study period. You will be prohibited from smoking through out your stay and until the last sample is collected.

- You should not consume any alcoholic product like beer, whisky, brandy, rum etc. at least 72 hours (3days) before the commencement of the study until the last sample collection is done.

- You should not take grapefruit products, xanthine containing foods or beverages like tea, coffee, chocolates, soft drinks etc. at least 72 hours (3days) before the commencement of the study and until the last sample is collected.

- The products mentioned above are likely to interfere with the action of medicines which is being tested and may give improper results. On admission day at our facility you will be thoroughly checked for the above mentioned prohibited items.

- If you have or ever had asthma or other lung disease, diabetes, severe allergies, heart or kidney disease, then you should tell our doctor at the facility about all these. The doctor at the facility will evaluate whether the XXX suspension can be given to you or not.

- You should not have participated in any other clinical research using experimental drug or had bled more than 350 ml in the past 3 months.

- You should tell our doctor at the facility if you plan to become pregnant or breast feeding (for female volunteers only).

- You should participate in the study only if you have not used any implanted or injected hormonal contraceptive during the past 6 months or taken oral hormonal contraceptives within 14 days before the study.

- Please present yourself on the admission day between 09.00 AM to 03.00 PM.

- You should be available to participate in the study as per the study schedule.

- In each period you have to fast overnight for 10 hours before consuming the high fat breakfast. If you are unable to meet this requirement, you will be discontinued from the study. After taking this medicine, you are required to fast for 5 hours.

- In each period of study, calculated quantity of the food will be served to you. It is very important that you consume the whole quantity of food that is served.

- You will be asked to fulfil other study requirements such as fluid restriction. You should not take any liquid before 01 hour and 01 hour after taking study medicine. Posture restriction (you must remain sitting for first 04 hours after taking medicine) and to limit physical activity through out your stay at our facility during study.

7. **Blood Collection:** In each period of study, a total of 23 blood samples will be collected using a flexible tube inserted into your blood vessel (intravenous cannula) or by venipuncture using a fresh needle each time of sampling. The blood sample will be collected as per the following schedule:

| Amount of blood collection | Sampling time in hours | Total number of samples |
|---|---|---|
| 4 ml at each sampling point | First two before 90 minutes of drug administration (0.00 hr) and the remaining at 0.25, 0.50, 0.75, 1.00, 1.25, 1.50, 1.75, 2.00, 2.50, 3.00, 3.50, 4.00, 5.00, 6.00, 8.00, 10.00, 12.00, 16.00, 24.00, 36.00 and 48.00 hr. | 23 |

The total volume collected per study participant in this study will not exceed 229 ml including the blood samples collection for screening, post clinical assessment of laboratory parameters and any additional or repeat tests.

8. **Possible Risks involved in the Study:** The drug that you are going to take is not a new drug. It is already available in the market and has undergone extensive clinical trials. However, the test medicine (new product of the available drug) is a new product that has not

been studied and the reference product is not new (it is already in the market).

It is important for you to take note of possibility of side effects due to medicine.  But they occur rarely after a single dose. The common side effects of the medicines that you are going to take are: -----, ---, -----, etc. They are temporary and reversible.

Kindly contact our physician in our laboratory for more details before signing the consent form.

The blood drawing procedure may cause pain, burning sensation or development of bruise at the site where the needle is placed to draw blood. This procedure may also occasionally cause light – headedness and fainting.  These reactions are usually of short duration, and limited to a feeling of being unwell, accompanied by sweating and a variation in heartbeats.

Only trained and qualified staff will perform the study procedures like taking blood samples. Medically trained staff will be available at all times to attend you and provide the necessary care. All the staff will take due care to reduce any risk that may occur to you. Additional medical care facility is available in case you do need.

9.  **Benefit to you and the Society:** You will get a medical check up free of cost (as given in section 3) and you will be informed of health status. You will be paid for your time and participation as per the section 10. If the test product is approved for marketing, the society will be benefited and you will have satisfaction of participation and contribution.

10.  **Payments:** You will be paid Rs. ----------/- for your time and participating in the study.  You will be paid an additional amount of Rs. --/- on full compliance to the study requirements. This cash payment will be made as per the schedule mentioned in the compensation section.  There will be a gap of 5 days between last blood sample collection of period II and final payment day.  In these 5 days, your health status, after completion of the study, will be assessed and you will be advised accordingly whether any changes in the laboratory investigation (value) requires attention.

In case you leave the study in mid way for any reason, ethics committee guidelines will be followed to make payments. This means that if you are dropped from the study due to study drug related effects or dropped because of protocol violations, you will be paid to the extent of your participation.

11. **Your Rights as a Volunteer:** Your participation in this study is purely voluntary and you are free to withdraw yourself from the study at any time.

    If you have any question during the study, or experience a side effect or research related injury, you are free to contact our following staff in the laboratory:

    1. **Dr. xxxxxx,** MD (Principal Investigator) at (Telephone Number).

    2. **Dr. yyyyy,** MD (Medical Investigator) at (Telephone Number).

    In case you experience any side effect related to study medicine or research related injury, proper medical care will be provided directly at our facility or will be facilitated by our organization with an insurance coverage for indemnity. This medical care will be free and will be at no cost to you.

    However, you will not be eligible to gain above benefit if you fail to follow all medical suggestions, instructions given to you and if you take any measures that can either cause or aggravate any kind of injury by yourself.

    Your rights as volunteer will be monitored by Independent Ethics Committee (IEC) which has approved this study. You may address your complaint and questions relating to your rights as a research participant to:

    Mr. zzzzzzz,

    Chairman, IEC,

    (Address and Telephone Numbers)

    Please give your unique code number assigned you when you contact the above persons.

12. **Confidentiality:** One unique code number is given to you as a participant of this study. Your records, photograph and finger print will identify you as a participant of the study. All records and test results will be attached with this code number to protect your identity. These records may be examined by the people who are working with the project, sponsor, Ethics Committee, and/or regulatory bodies. Any personal identifier in the study documents will be removed before the data is shared, published or processed by any third party.

    With the signing this document, you are enrolled to take part in this study and you allow us to make your records available to the people who are working in the project, sponsor, Ethics Committee and Regulatory bodies. However, it is voluntary for you to decide whether to sign this document and participate in the study or not. It is your decision.

**We, at (Name of the organization), appreciate and thank you for showing interest to participate in this research study.**

13. **Consent Form for Volunteer Participation in this Study:**

*STUDY TITLE: Single Dose Fasting Bioequivalence Study of XXX (name of the product with strength and manufacturer) to XXX (name of the product with strength and manufacturer) in Healthy Adult Male Volunteers.*

**Protocol Number and Version:**

I have been informed to my satisfaction that:

- My participation in this study is voluntary.
- This study provides me no medical benefits other than a medical check up.
- My blood samples collected during screening will be subjected for analysis in different stages. My eligibility in one stage will make me suitable for the next. In case abnormalities are noticed in any stage, my samples will not be processed for further analysis and my blood samples will be disposed off.
- I have the rights to be provided with answers to questions arising during the course of the study.
- I can withdraw from the study at any time without prejudice to future medical care or selection for future studies.
- My study participation can be terminated by (Name of the organization) at any time if I violate the study protocol or to protect my health.
- The Principal Investigator, in consultation with sponsor, reserves the right to terminate the study for safety reasons at any time or any other rational reason.
- I will receive a copy of the signed consent form.

**Further more I declare that:**

- My date of birth is ---------- and I am 18 – 45 years old.
- I have read and understood this information sheet dated ---and had opportunity to ask questions.

- I understand that my participation in this study is voluntary and I am free to withdraw at any time, without assigning any reason, without my medical care or legal rights being affected.

- I currently require no medical treatment or care.

- I have not participated in any experimental studies conducted at this organization (Name the organization) or any other place in the past three months.

- I do not have any objections on my data being used for scientific purpose(s). However, I understand that my identity will not be revealed in any information released to third parties or published.

- I will comply with all administrative requirements of this organization (name of the organization).

I, -------------------, have received a copy of this form. The details have been explained to me by the staff of ----(name of the organization) and I have understood the same. I hereby willingly affix my signature in confirmation of my participation in this study.

-----------------------------

(Volunteer Signature and Date)

-------------------------

--------------------------------------

(Consent obtained by)

(Signature and Date)

I confirm that the subject can read and has fully understood the procedure and risks associated with the participation in this study.

----------------------------------

(Signature of Study Physician and Date)

## SCHEDULE

**The following schedule will be observed for the study:**

**(Include the date of study too.)**

| Period I and II | | |
|---|---|---|
| **Day** | **Time** | **Activity** |
| **Day – 1 (previous day to dosing) period I** | 9.00 am to 3.00 pm | Checking into the Lab. (name the organization) |
| | 10.00 am onwards | Urine sample collection for testing drugs of abuse |
| | 2.00 pm | Lunch |
| | 8.00 pm | Dinner (standard low fat meal) |
| | 9.30 pm | Bed time |
| **DOSING DAY for period I** | 6.00 to 7.28 am | Vital Check up |
| | 6.30 am to 7. 58 am | Blood sample collection before consumption of study medicine |
| | 7.30 am | High fat breakfast |
| | 8.00 am | Drug administration and blood sampling at 0.00 hrs. |
| | 8.15 am | 0.25 hrs sampling |
| | 8.30 am | 0.50 hrs sampling |
| | 8.45 am | 0.75 hrs sampling |
| | 9.00 am | 1.00 hrs sampling |
| | 9.25 am | 1.25 hrs sampling |
| | 9.30 am | 1.50 hrs sampling |
| | 9.45 am | 1.75 hrs sampling |
| | 10.00 am | 2.00 hrs sampling |
| | 10.30 am | 2.50 hrs sampling |
| | 11.00am | 3.00 hrs sampling |
| | 11.30 am | 3.5 hrs sampling |
| | 12.00 noon | 4.00 hrs sampling |
| | 1.00 pm | 5.00 hrs sampling and Lunch |
| | 2.00 pm | 6.00 hrs sampling |
| | 4.00 pm | 8.00 hrs sampling |
| | 5.00 pm | Snacks |
| | 6.00 pm | 10.00 hrs sampling |

| | 8.00 pm | 12.00 hrs sampling |
| --- | --- | --- |
| | 9.00 pm | Dinner |
| | 9.30 pm | Bed time |
| | 12.00 night | 16.00 hrs sampling |
| **Day +1 (next day of dosing day) for period I** | 8.00 am | 24.00 hrs sampling and breakfast |
| | 1.00 pm | Lunch |
| | 5.00 pm | Snacks |
| | 8.00 pm | 36.00 hrs sampling |
| | 9.00 pm | Dinner |
| | 9.30 pm | Bed time |
| **Day +2 (two days after dosing day) for period I** | 8.00 am | 48 hrs sampling and breakfast |
| | 8.30 am onwards | Check out |
| **Day +2 (two days after dosing day) for period II** | 08.00 am | 48 hrs sampling and breakfast followed by post clinical check up |
| | 8.30 am onwards | Study Exit |

**There will be gap of 07 days between each period.**

**COMPENSATION**

| Details of Compensation | Amount in Rupees | Payment Schedule |
| --- | --- | --- |
| **Study participation compensation** | **5000/-** | On Dosing day + 2 of period II: 2000/- On Dosing Day + 7 of period II: 3000/- |
| ***Compliance Incentive (on compliance to the study requirements for all periods)** | **1500/-** | On the final payment day (Dosing day + 7of period II) (post clinical assessment and payment) |
| **Total** | **6500/-** | |

* if you are found to be in compliance to the study related requirements (including on time arrival to the facility and comply with all other study requirements mentioned in information sheet) during the study, you will be eligible for this compliance incentive.

# CONTRACT RESEARCH ORGANIZATIONS (CRO) WITH CONTACT DETAILS

| Sl. No. | Name of the Company | Address | E. mail and website |
|---|---|---|---|
| 1 | Accutest Research Laboratories (I) Pvt. Ltd. | A-31, MIDC, TTC, Ind. Area, Khairne, Navi Mumbai- 400709 | Email : accutest @ vsnl.net<br>www.accutestindia.com |
| 2 | Ace Biomed Pvt. Ltd. Indian Cork Mill Compound, | Sakhi - Vihar Road, Powai, Mumbai - 400072, India | Email : info@acebiomed.com<br>www.acebiomed.com |
| 3 | Actimus Biosciences Pvt. Ltd | 4th Floor, Varun Towers, Kasturba Marg Siripuram, Visakhapatnam - 530003, India | Email : queries@actimusbio.com<br>www.actimusbio.com |
| 4 | Apothecaries Ltd | 579 Devli East Sanik Farms, New Delhi, 110062 | Email : cro@apothecaries.net<br>www.apothecaries.net |
| 5 | Asian Clinical Trials | 5/F Screne Chambers, Road - 7, Banjara Hills Hyderabad 500034 | Email : vsunder@act.india.com |
| 6 | Aurigene Discovery Technologies | Electronic City, Phase II, 39, 40 Electronic City Phase II, Housur Road, KIADB Industrial Area, Banglore, 560100 | Email : partnerships@aurigene.com<br>www.aurigene.com |
| 7 | Avra Laboratories | Avra House, 54, Sai Enclave, Habsiguda, Hyderabad - 500007 | Email : info@avralab.com,<br>www.avralab.com |
| 8 | Bioserve Biotechnologies (I) Pvt. Ltd | Lab No. 8, ICICI Knowledge park, Genome Valley, Turkapalli Village, Shameerpet Mandal, Hyderabad - 500078 | Email : info@bioserve.com,<br>www.bioserve.com |

| 9 | Chembiotek Research International | Block BN, Sector V, Salt Lake City, Kolkata - 700091 | Email : research@chembiotek.com, www.chembiotek.com |
|---|---|---|---|
| 10 | Clinigene International | 20th KM, Hosur Road Electronic City Banglore 560100 (India | Email : contact.us@biocon.com, http://www.biocon.com |
| 11 | Clininvent Research Pvt. Ltd | A-302, Everest Chambers Next to Star TV office, Marol Naka Andheri - kurla Road, Andheri (E) Mumbai- 400059, India | Email : arunbhatt@clininvent.com, www.clinvent.com |
| 12 | Clin Tec India International Pvt. Ltd. | No. 104, IInd Cross, Ramaiah Reddy Layout, Benson Cross, Benson Town, Banglore - 560046 | Email : india@clintec.com, www.clintec.com |
| 13 | Clintrac International Pvt. Ltd | IIIrd Floor, East II, Vydehi Hospital - 82 IPIP Area, Whitefield Road, Banglore - 560066 | email : info@clintracinternational.com www.clintracintl.com |
| 14 | D & O CRO | 108, Sundaram Estate, Of. BKSD Road, Govandi (E) Mumbai - 88 | Email : info@dnogroup.com www.dnogroup.com |
| 15 | Dr. Reddy's Laboratories Limited | 7-1-27, Ameerpet, Hyderabad 500016, India | Email : webmaster@ddreddys.com www.ddreddys.com |
| 16 | Eli Lilly and company (India) Pvt. Ltd | Plot - 92, Sector 32, Industrial Area Gurgaon - 122001, Haryana | Email : lillyindia@lilly.com www.lillyindia.co.in |
| 17 | Glaxosmithkline Pharmaceuticals Limited | Dr. Annie Besant Road, Worli, Mumbai - 400025 | Email : askus@gsk.com www.gsk-india.com |

*Table contd...*

| 18 | Gokula Metro Polis Clinical Laboratories Pvt. Ltd | M.S. Ramaiah Memorial Hospital New Bel Road, MSRIT Post, Banglore - 560094 | Email : gokula@metropolisindia.com |
|---|---|---|---|
| 19 | GVK Biosciences Pvt. Ltd | 210, My Home Tycoon, 6-3-1192, Kundanbagh Begumpet, Hyderabad - 500016(AP | www.gvkbio.com |
| 20 | iGATE Clinical Research International Private Limited | 101-102, Alpha, Hiranandani Gardns Powai, Mumbai, 400076 | Email : infoicri@igate.com www.igate.com/icri |
| 21 | Intas Pharmaceuticals | Chinubhai Center, Off. Nehru Bridge Ashram Road, Ahmedabad - 09 | www. info@intaspharma.com intasbiopharma.co.in |
| 22 | International Tech Park Ltd | Discover , 9th Floor, Unit III Whitefield Road , Banglore - 560066 | Email : pramod@avesthagen.com http://aquasltd.com |
| 23 | INTOX Private | 375, Urawade, Pirangut Taluda Mulshi District - Pune, 412108 | Email : intox@vsnl.com, www.intoxlab.com |
| 24 | Kendle India | 23-24, Vatika Business Center, 2nd Floor First India Place, Block B, Mehrauli - Gurgaon Road Sushant Lok - I Gurgaon - 02, U.P | Email : doshi.bharat@kendle.com www.kendle.com |
| 25 | Lambda Therapeutic Research Ltd | 42, Premier House I, Bodakdev, Sarkhej Gandhinagar Highway Ahmedabad 380054, Gujarat | Email : ahmedabad@lambda-cro.com www. lambda-cro.com |

**Table** *contd...*

| | | | |
|---|---|---|---|
| 26 | Lotus Labs Pvt/ Ltd. | 582, KC A Enclave, 8th Block Koramangala Banglore - 560095 | Email : info@lotuslabs.com www.lotuslabs.com |
| 27 | Lupin Limited | Laxmi Towers, "B" Wing, 4th Floor Bandra Kurla complex, Mumbai - 400051 | Email : api@lupinworld.com www.lupinworld.com |
| 28 | Magene Life Science | Research Centre, D No. 14-59/3 Pudur Post Raval Kole X Roads, Medchal Mandal, Hyderabad - 501401 | Email : info@magenelifesciences.com www.magenelifesciences.com |
| 29 | Manipal Acunova | Manipal Towers 14, Airport Road Banglore- Karnataka- 560100 | Email : nivedita.shenoy@acunovalife.com www.acunovalife.com |
| 30 | Matrix laboratories limited | 1-1-11/1, 4th Floor, Sai Ram Towers Alexander Road, Secunderabad - 500003 | Email : matrix@matrixlabsindia.com www.matrixlabsindia.com |
| 31 | Metropolis Clinical Laboratories | 250 - D Udyog Bhawan, Hind Cycle Marg Behind Glaxo, Worli, Mumbai - 400030 | Email : support@metropolisindia.com www.metropolisindia.com |
| 32 | Novo Noordisk India Private Limited | 8th Floor, Raheja Towers, East Wing 26/27, M.G.Road, Banglore, Karnatka - 560001 | Email : investigators@omnicarecr.com www.omnicarecr.com |
| 33 | Pharma - Olam International | 217, 4th Cross, 19th Main Koramangala 6th Block, Banglore - 95 | Email : info@pharm-olam.com, www.pharm-olam.com |
| 34 | Pharmanet | Unit 1101, level 11, Millenia Tower B 1&2 Murphy Road, Ulsoor, Banglore - 560008 | www.pharmanet.com |

*Table Contd...*

| | | | |
|---|---|---|---|
| 35 | PPD pharmaceutical Development India | 801-804, Powai plaza Hiranandani Business park Powai , Mumbai - 400076 | |
| 36 | Quintitles Technologies (India ) private Limited | Brigade South parade, 3rd Floor, 10, M.G.Road, Bangalore – 560001 | Email : india@quintiles.com www.quintiles.com |

# USEFUL WEBSITES

1. Central Drugs Standard Control Organization (CDSCO): www.cdsco.nic.in

2. Council for International Organizations of Medical Sciences (CIOMS): http://www.cioms.ch/

3. European Agency for Evaluation of Medical Products (EMEA): www.emea.europa.eu/

4. Indian Council for Medical Research (ICMR): http://www. icmr.nic.in

5. International Conference on Harmonization (ICH): http://www. ich.org

6. US Food and Drug Administration (USFDA): http:// www.fda.gov

7. World Health Organization (WHO): www.who.int

8. World Health Organization Country Office for India (WHO-India): www.whoindia.org

9. World Medical Association (WMA): http://www.wma.net

10. World Trade Organization: http://www.wto.org

# References

1. A Bitter Pill – WEMOS, December 2007.

2. Accreditation Standards for Clinical Trials: Ethics Committee, Investigator and Clinical Trial Sites, National Accreditation Board for Hospitals (NABH), First Draft, 2014.

3. Anuradha Kulkarni and Arun Bhat, Indian Regulations and Patient Safety during Clinical Trials – An Analysis, Pharma Times, 47(8), August 2015.

4. Binny Krishnakutty, Shantala Bellary, Naveen BR Kumar, and Latha S Moodahadu, Data management in clinical research: An overview, Indian Journal of Pharmacology, 44(2), March-April 2012.

5. Bio Business Summit, "Global Clinical Trials in India – Prospects and Challenges", White Paper by FICCI and Cygnus, 2005.

6. Conference on Clinical Research: Road Map for India, Background Paper, 2003.

7. Contemporary Ethical Issues in Biomedical and Health Research, ICMR, New Delhi, 2007.

8. D. Sreedhar et al, Clinical Trials in India: Current Scenario and Future outlook, The Pharma Review, May 2009.

9. Drugs and Cosmetics Act and the Rules, Government of India, CDSCO website, http://cdsco.nic.in , accessed on 15th January 2010.

10. Drugs and Cosmetics Rules 1945, as amended till 15th August 2013.

11. Ethical Guidelines for Biomedical Research on Human Participants, Indian Council of Medical Research, New Delhi, 2006.

12. First Round Up of Developments in the Pharmaceutical Sector, Department of Pharmaceuticals, Government of India, 2008.

13. G. P. Mohanta, P. K. Manna and G. Gayatri, Placebo Controlled Clinical Trials & Ethical Concerns, Chronicle Pharmabiz, 61st IPC Issue, December 10, 2009.

14. Good Clinical Practice for Clinical Research in India, http://cdsco.nic.in/html/GCP1.html ; accessed on 29.11.2009.

15. Guidelines for Bioavailability & Bioequivalence Studies, CDSCO, Government of India, March 2005.

16. Guidelines for Responsible Data Management in Scientific Research, Developed by Clinical Tools, Inc.,

17. Guidelines for Writing Standard Operating Procedures for Clinical Trials – Instruction Manual, CDSCO, 2005.

18. Handbook for Good Clinical Research Practice (GCP), WHO, 2005.

19. Health Research Methodology: A Guide for Training in Research Methods, Second Edition, WHO Regional Office for Western Pacific, Manila, 2001.

20. Johan PE Karlberg and Marjorie A Speers (Editors), Reviewing Clinical Trials: A Guide for Ethics Committee, Karlberg, Johan Petter Einar, 2010.

21. Joseph Millum, David Wendler, Ezekiel J. Emanuel, The 50th Anniversary of the Declaration of Helsinki Progress but Many Remaining Challenges, JAMA,;310(20):2143-2144, 2013.

22. Management of Safety Information from Clinical Trials, Report of CIOMS Working Group VI, Geneva, 2005.

23. Ohmann *et al,* Standard requirements for GCP-compliant data management in multinational clinical trials, Trials, 12(85), 2011.

24. Raman Sehgal, Outsourcing Clinical Trials in India – Opportunities and Challenges, The Pharma Review, May 2009.

25. Report of the Professor Ranjit Roy Chaudhury Expert Committee to Formulate Policy and Guidelines for Approval of New Drugs, Clinical Drugs and Banning of Drugs, Government of India, 2013.

26. Sandhya Srinivasan, Ethical Concern in Clinical Trials in India: an Investigation, Centre for Studies in Ethics and Rights, Mumbai, February 2009.

27. Subhash C. Mandal and Maitreyee Mandal, Evolution of Regulation for Conducting Clinical Trials in India, Pharma Times, August 2009.

28. WHO Expert Committee on Specifications for Pharmaceutical Preparations, Fortieth report, World Health Organization, Geneva, 2006.

# Index